MW01278462

Sleeping For Pilots
& Cabin Crew
(and other Insomniacs)

by
An Anonymous
Airbus A380 Captain

ISBN 978-0-9944760-1-2
Paperback

'Trying to study for the simulator but made the fatal mistake of uploading *"Sleeping For Pilots & Cabin Crew"* onto my kindle!

I cannot put it down and **laughing out loud** at some anecdotes ...

Every shift worker needs this book!'

' ... as entertaining as Bill Bryson's books I reckon! '

-- C.J. Boeing 777 Captain

Essential Reading For Aircrew
(& anyone else working the backside of the clock)!

I gave up a career that I loved, in large part because the night shifts, and subsequent fatigue, were killing me.

Had this informative, well researched, and humorous book been available, **I might still be flying.**

-- I.H. (former) A380 Captain

It is always the **original ideas that win** with books, and this is one that **most people have been waiting** for someone to write.

It's very well-researched and well-written; **deserves to be read.**

- Navjot Singh, Author & Photo-Journalist

National Library Of Australia

Cataloguing-in-Publication Entry

Author	An Anonymous Airbus A380 Captain: J.C.N.
Title	Sleeping For Pilots & Cabin Crew (And Other Insomniacs)
ISBN	978-0-9944760-1-2 (pbk)
Subjects	- - Sleeping - - Air Pilots - - - - Cabin Crew - - Health - - - - Insomnia - - Travel - - - - Anecdotes
Dewey	TBA
Publisher	www ProfessionalSleeping com Al Ghozlan 4, Street 5, The Greens, U.A.E 219 Bridport Street West, Albert Park, 3206 Australia
Printed by	CreateSpace, An Amazon.com Company
Typeface	MinionPro 12 point
BISAC	Health & Fitness / Sleep & Sleep Disorders
Cover Design	Clarrie Wilkinson, Bird Rock Productions
Cover Photographs	©JamesNixon.com

Boring (But Important)
Legal Stuff

The author and publisher of this book and the accompanying materials have used their best efforts in preparing this book. The information contained in this book is for educational purposes. Therefore, if you wish to apply ideas contained in this book, you are taking full responsibility for your actions.

Examples in these materials are not to be interpreted as a promise or guarantee of successful sleep.

The author and publisher do not warrant the performance, effectiveness or applicability of sites listed or linked to in this book.

All links are for information purposes only and are not warranted for content, accuracy or other implied or explicit purpose.

Email **contact@professionalsleeping.com**

Table of Contents

Dedication

Vale Jim Jacobs

A pleasure flying with you.

Foreword

Who Needs This Book?

Anyone who is going to sit next to me.

My first real airline job saw me, as First Officer, doing a walk around in the cold and dark before sunrise. The international airport was coming to life. The darkness of the western sky was punctuated by landing lights of the transcontinental "red eye" which became an airliner and soon a noisy one, as the first reversers of the day crackled in the pre-dawn chill. Nowhere in my imaginings did I think one day I would be sitting in the cockpit of that plane. I thought people slept at night.

Well, *people* do. Pilots, Cabin Crew and Engineers don't.

All my dreams came true when Graeme Stafford rang and offered me a job flying the Boeing 727, the sexiest looking plane in the world (besides the Concorde). It had three engines and three cockpit crew, one of whom was a Flight Engineer. Our fleet, dwindling because they were old and soon banned for making too much noise, had a number of passenger planes and two freighters. Freighters, I learned, flew at night and always smelt of horse-urine.

Specialized skills were handed down from the Flight Engineers to the junior First Officers: how to run the galley and make the coffee and sleep during the day. Unlike the United States where they had junior pilots running the Flight Engineer's panel, we had career engineers. Most had twenty years' experience working on the 727 in the hangar, the majority as back-of-clock shift workers.

On the first triple-night freighter pairing I learned the tricks of how to sleep in hotel rooms when the rest of the world was up and awake, and banging against the skirting-boards of the room next door with vacuum cleaners. These tricks weren't passed on because they were nice guys. It was because they would be sitting right behind us if we crashed the plane due to fatigue. As a great Australian Prime Minister said:

'In the race of life, always back self-interest.
At least you know it's trying.'

Our Flight Engineers wanted us to be alert when it counted, and they taught us the tricks.

You might soon be sitting beside me as we fly the Airbus A380 across half the planet in one flight, or you may be my cabin crew. I want you to be as well-rested as possible before we commit aviation, and I want to hand down the information that I was given by my mentors: the Flight Engineers.

Sadly, you will never fly with one. And that is your loss, for these guys were salt of the earth, our protectors, our friends, our wingmen, our teachers, our defenders; our mates. When female pilots arrived, they became brothers and the champions of the new era. They saved our lives in the air and, on layovers, shepherded us away from the nastiest strip clubs and helped get us back to the hotel when walking was a challenge. One was so proud that I had made it to the big time, he produced a postcard and made me write to my Mum on my first layover in Kings Cross Sydney. I failed to notice that the picture was of a transvestite stripper until I went to my parents for a family dinner a few weeks later and saw it on the fridge. Even then I couldn't decipher what I had written on the back.

One made me pause as we attempted to get a senior captain out of a bar in which a drunken lady had taken a shine to him. Her husband had arrived and was annoyed that the skipper refused to "spend an hour" with her:

'What's wrong with you? Isn't my wife good enough for you?!'

Thinking I was in a bad movie, I marveled at how fast the Flight Engineer paid our tab and was getting us out of there. He blurted:

'We gotta go now, I don't wanna spend ANOTHER night in jail on a layover...'

Talk about burying the lead story. As I downed my glass I spluttered,

'You've been in jail on a layover?'

By this time he had the skipper by the arm and was propelling him out the door.

'Twice,' he said over his shoulder.

Someone should write a book about them all.

o 0 o

This book consists of everything I have learned about sleeping in my thirty years of flying. Getting control of your sleep right now is the only way you can turn this job into a long-term career.

I have divided this book in two parts. The first is an analysis of the many variables that can affect your sleep. The second part is the 'how-to' section. These tips and tricks have been tested in the laboratory of life. They work under the harshest conditions in the world: the *moving sleep cycle* of the flight crew. Like no-one else does it.

Fire fighters, police, doctors, nurses, shift workers all get a roster that allows a sign-on at the same time for up to six days in a row. They feel like crap, but they can get a routine going. We rise with the sun, fly to a location, arrive in the late afternoon, have twenty-two hours off then fly back overnight, arriving before the sun rises on day three. On day four we sign on in the afternoon and fly until midnight. And so on. If we are travelling east and west then jet lag adds to the mix.

There are entire industries trying to sell you things to sleep faster, better, easier, softer and longer. Few of them work. Some are outright dangerous and can put your flight crew license at risk, not to mention the lives of your passengers. I have trawled through hundreds of websites and research papers to support the suggestions I offer in this book. Each one is listed in the footnotes so you can check the latest information. I have not knowingly plagiarized any work. I have quoted slabs and given attribution where appropriate. Don't think I am a doctor or a scientist. I am a writer who became a pilot who has only ever slept in once. Thinking about that day makes my blood run cold twenty years later.

A few organizations need mentioning, if only because they are a great resource if you ever need information.

The Mayo Clinic[1] should be regarded as not only a legitimate source of information, but the jewel in the crown of medical research and patient care in the world. Since 1864 it has grown from a humble medical practice into the Nobel Prize winning organization we see today: the first clinic to specialize in aviation medicine. Their website should be your first stop to get unbiased, up-to-date information.

The Harvard Medical School and the Harvard Health Publications[2] are another good resource. I have not read their studies in relation to sleep during the writing of this book, for fear of stealing their work, but I may have read a few of their articles a few years ago. Their website offers well-researched articles on health issues and is the best way to get educated in a hurry.

The United Nations Children's Fund (UNICEF[3]) and The World Health Organization (WHO[4]) are the best sources to provide information about wide-scale public health issues.

When I lived in Vietnam during the first bird-flu outbreak in 2003 we kept asking someone at our hotel to read the WHO website, which declared that we could still eat cooked eggs for breakfast. Too late; all the eggs had been destroyed.

WebMD[5] and Drugs[6] are two quick websites to find out about individual issues. Don't trust your memory when it comes to taking medication.

Google, Wikipedia[7] and Google Scholar[8] are often the starting points in my research.

This is the book you would have written if you had interviewed a few thirty-year veterans and spent about a year of your days-off trolling through the published research papers, newspaper and magazine stories and websites. I have tried to distill some heavy topics into light reading; and can guarantee that if you do everything I suggest, you will get control of your sleep and sleep better than you've ever slept before. If not, I will give you your money back.

If there is a chance your issues are medical, do not believe a word of what is written here. Get yourself to a doctor, one specializing in sleep issues. For other issues, obesity for example, get a team together of your doctor and a specialist: a dietitian maybe, and even a physiotherapist.

That is the essence of piloting. We are trained problem-solvers and we work on the motto that a problem-shared is a problem-solved. Your body is more intricate and has far more computing power than my A380. If, like an airplane, it's not running as advertised by the manufacturer, get help.

A great man, Ted Whitten, who was suffering terminal cancer said:

'No-one knows how long the nights are ...'

His words stuck with me for all these years and I vowed to share the sleep tips that are about tricking your brain.

As an anonymous comic pointed out in 2013:

'Sleeping is the only thing you do, where you have to pretend you're doing it ... in order to do it'.

Let me know how you go by emailing me. I can't wait to get your feedback.

Sleep well.

The Anonymous A380 Captain
November 2015

From the Logbook

The term *"sleep like a baby"* is adult speak for sleeping well. In actual fact, most babies seem to sleep for about three hours before waking up in their own excreta, screaming.

Part One

Things that affect your sleep

Alcohol

All of us have, at some point, experienced the problem of having too much alcohol during an overnight or layover. How often have you woken up with the repetitive Sky News music blaring from the TV in a brightly-lit hotel room with the remnants of a club sandwich and fries mashed into the side of your face and pillow?

It's okay. We've all done it ... once.

But that doesn't mean it's clever, and it sure doesn't help you sleep well. Alcohol has the ability to produce a fast-acting sedative sleep; you will go out like a light and sleep solidly for about one or two hours. You'll even sleep through the room service doorbell and fire alarms. But it's not proper sleep and you never get the Rapid Eye Movement (REM) sleep necessary to restore human cells.

It also makes you dehydrated, which means you will wake feeling like crap, with a headache. So it's best not to get drunk if restful sleep is your aim. Two glasses of wine with dinner interspersed with a glass of water will have no effect and help you relax and sleep after flight. Any more than a couple of drinks is not going to help you sleep. Binge drinking is a problem within the airline industry. Employees are prevented from drinking for so long before their next flight, that they feel a need to down a number of drinks in a short time while they can. It is a self-defeating exercise.

Aviation legislation has two prongs worth noting. The first: pilots call *"Bottle-To-Throttle,"* describes the number of hours between the last drink and the start of the next duty period which varies between eight and twelve hours. The second is the catch-all clause: you may not enter an aircraft for the purposes of duty - even paxing - under the effects of alcohol or drugs. This means that while you may have stopped drinking in time, your body may have not metabolized the alcohol if you were on a binge. You have to keep track of the number of drinks and work out how long you need.

As a rough guide, three standard units of alcohol in the first hour brings your BAC (Blood Alcohol Concentration) to 0.05, and one standard unit per hour will keep you there. Then you need to one hour to metabolize each 0.1. This means that in the bar after a flight you have four standard drinks in two hours, you will need at least six hours before you are back to 0.0, and double that time just to be safe. If you walk onto your next flight twelve hours after your last drink, you should pass the random test. The threat is when you are not in a bar, where each unit is measured. At dinner parties there is a tendency to use huge glasses and fill them to a satisfying level, increasing the amount consumed.

If restful sleep is your aim, cut back on the grog.

RECAPPING:

- **Binge drinking is a problem in the airline industry.**
- **Try to monitor your consumption.**
- **Introduce a glass of water between drinks.**
- **Allow adequate time for the alcohol to leave your system.**
- **If restful sleeping is your aim, stop the alcohol after two glasses.**

From The Logbook

Three rooms at the Canberra Hyatt hotel are almost underground. Someone told the Cabin Crew that they were haunted - true story - and their union arranged that they never had to stay in them. So the three rooms became the province of the Captain, First Officer and Flight Engineer of the last nightly airplane into Canberra, a Boeing 727. One particular Captain arrived in his room over-refreshed after a long session in the lobby bar and decided to take a pre-sleep shower.

He awoke to find one of Canberra's finest Rescue Fire Fighters reaching over him to turn off the shower tap. Slumped on the floor of the shower with his bum sealed over the drain, the water poured on and on as he snored the house down. When the water reached a significant depth, flooding out into the hallway and into the other two rooms, the alarm was raised.

Ever since he has gone by the nickname: *"Plugger."*

Bed Bugs

For a time in the summer of 2010 there were bed bugs in every hotel room in New York City, or so the media would have you believe. There must have been something in it, for an internet search shows how serious the city fathers have taken it[9]. As an aircrew you can expect to meet up with bed bugs during your career. Here is all you need to know.

Bed bugs are real. They hide during the day and come out between 10 p.m. and 6 a.m. They travel about three meters (ten feet) to feed on, wait for it, *human blood* then return to chill with their mates. They find their host, like mosquitoes, by sniffing for carbon dioxide. They are also believed to be attracted to pheromones. Bed bugs can last without a feed from 20 to 400 days. They prefer to live within one and half meters (five feet) of their meals.

They can't stand heat above 45 Celsius (113 Fahrenheit) or exposure to freezing temperatures of -16 Celsius (3 Fahrenheit) for an hour or more. Steaming for a prolonged time gets them too, at 65-75 Celsius (150-170 Fahrenheit); as you are already thinking, the cure may be uncomfortable for the host too. And what are you pointing the steam iron at?

Oh, another way of getting them is to set fire to the room.

Crevices, drapes, behind pictures, wallpaper, even electrical plugs, any sneaky hiding spot you can imagine is where you'll find them. Mattresses, bed bases and headboards are their ideal location. Fabric, wood and paper hiding spots are best; they are less happy with metal. Females can lay roughly twelve eggs a day, and they live from a year to eighteen months.

Why would they hurt you?

It makes no sense to have you get sick or die. In an ideal world you'd keep providing the nourishment every night and remain nice and healthy.

Which is how it is, mostly.

When you are asleep, they arrive and bite you, injecting an anesthetic and an anticoagulant so you don't feel it or find bloody blotches as evidence. Within three minutes, up to ten for a mature adult, they are done and it's off back to their hiding spot to put their six feet up and digest dinner. You may notice the bite marks but will be hard pressed to tell the difference between it and a mosquito or tiny spider bite, except that there is no red dot in the middle of the inflamed area. Some people have allergic reactions to their bites but it's rare. Nature provides that it is good for business for the host to continue the free ride. More than likely someone would excessively scratch an itchy bite, leading to infection. Dab bite marks with an antiseptic cream.

Do they carry disease?

They have been known to be exposed to up to twenty-eight diseases, one study says forty-five, but after one hundred years of research bed bugs have *never* transmitted diseases to humans. Compared to mosquitoes, they are nature's gentlemen.

How do they get around?

In your luggage. Since the advent of the airplane bed bugs have become the eternal travelers. Never, ever, place your suitcase on a bed. Hotels have frames that you unfold and on which you place your suitcase. Make sure it is not touching the wall. Do not *ever* use the drawers in hotels and be suspicious of the wardrobes. Keep your packed clothes and shoes in plastic bags. Have extra plastic bags. Sort dirty clothes into separate bags for washing when you get home.

What do they look like?

They are egg-shaped flat insects with six legs, the front ones bent forward and the rest pointing rearwards. Bed bugs are light brown in color and about 4.5mm ($1/6^{th}$ inch) long and 2.5mm ($1/10^{th}$ inch) wide. Their eggs look like a grain of rice and are 2.5mm ($1/10^{th}$ inch) long and coated with a sticky substance.

How do I find them?

Good luck. Large infestations smell like "rotting raspberries." Have you any idea what that smells like? I wouldn't have a clue. Since the humble puppy's sense of smell can function in parts per trillion, it follows that you could train dogs to find them. And Americans do. Well trained, the success rate with bed bug sniffing pooches is approaching 80%. For the aircrew it's tricky taking a dog on every layover. You're better off with a torch and knowing where to find the usual suspects. The internet has hundreds of sites to help you, like the New York City website detailed in the footnotes[10]. I saved their diagram to Evernote and can look at it on my iPad whenever I need to search.

Getting rid of them.

Vacuuming works for the ones you can see, along the seam of the mattress or headboard, but professional help is needed if your room is infected. Expect the pest controller to make up to three visits. Maybe that's why room attendants always bang their vacuum cleaners against the wall of every adjoining room when I try to sleep during the day. They are trying to dislodge house guests.

Bombing the rooms with chemicals isn't recommended. The amount of chemical needed to get into the crevices where the bugs live would kill the homeowner. And pesticides only work where you can see the blighters. You can get fabric mattress protectors in which you seal your mattress and base, preventing the bugs from escaping. Then there are 'cups' in which you place the feet of the bed to prevent the bugs clambering up or down, acting as a moat.

The leaves of Kidney Bean plants have tiny hairs that trap bed bugs' feet (I'm not kidding), so if you scatter these all around you may wake up to find your miniature vampires trapped amongst the greenery. Scientists are busy making synthetic tiny hooks which mimic the effect.

Any clothes or bedding that has been exposed to bugs has to be washed in hot water for at least thirty minutes at 60 Celsius (86 Fahrenheit). This kills all bugs in all stages of the life cycle. So will thirty minutes in the high cycle of a clothes drier for clothing that doesn't have to be washed.

When you return home from a layover, do not put your suit case on your bed. Take the dirty clothes (which are in a plastic bag, aren't they?) straight to the washing machine.

Dr. Joe says that they can be asphyxiated by putting your affected clothes in black bin bags, tied-up to prevent any oxygen getting-in. His inner murderer causing his eyes to sparkle, he continued:

"Use two bags, one inside the other. They're dead after three days. Easy!"

Become an expert at bed bug control.

If you find bed bugs, and you have been watching CSI, you can collect them using some adhesive tape. Bag 'em and present them to the hotel manager and your company. I'd take a few pictures instead.

How does it affect your sleep?

Even though the actual visitation of the bed bugs is designed by nature to be a benign experience, and they have never been known to transmit disease to humans, there is a psychological impact which sometimes causes insomnia. For me, having written this, and you, the reader, one thing is for certain: *neither of us is going to sleep well tonight as we dream about our little vampire friends crawling over our faces.*

RECAPPING:

- **Bed bugs are real.**
- **Study-up on how to spot evidence of bed bugs and learn how to scan your hotel rooms on arrival. Call the hotel manager on duty (MOD), complain and change rooms.**
- **They hide during the day and are active between 10 p.m. and 6 a.m.**
- **They travel about three meters (ten feet) to feed on human blood.**
- **They prefer to live within one and half meters (five feet) of their meals.**

- They find their host by sniffing for carbon dioxide.
- Bed bugs can last without a feed from 20 to 400 days.
- They arrive and bite you, injecting an anesthetic and an anticoagulant so you don't feel it or find evidence.
- Within three minutes, up to ten for a mature adult, they are done.
- After one hundred years of research bed bugs have never transmitted diseases to humans.
- They travel in luggage.
- Never, ever, place your suitcase on a bed.
- Instead use the frame provided and make sure it is not touching the wall.
- Do not *ever* use the drawers in hotels and be suspicious of the wardrobes.
- Keep your suitcase closed as much as possible.
- Put dirty clothes in plastic bags.
- When you return home, do not put your suitcase on your bed.
- Unpack your suitcase next to your washing machine.
- Any clothes or bedding that has been exposed to bugs has to be washed in hot water for at least thirty minutes at 60 Celsius (86 Fahrenheit), OR
- Sealed-up in plastic bags so no oxygen can get in for three days.

Body Clock

Central to learning how to sleep on demand is to become in touch with your body. This requires an understanding of your circadian rhythm, which is the twenty-four hour cycle of the planet as it revolves around its axis, whist trudging along its eternal (we hope) orbit of our favorite star. Diurnal variation means a twelve hour cycle and relates to tides, temperature maximum and minimum, and even air pressure.

If you are inclined, there are hundreds of books and scientific papers worth perusing, but you can take it as gospel that the earth and its inhabitants work on cycles. You can either work in ignorance, bumbling your way through life, or you can study yours and get it to work with you to help make your life easier.

90 Minute Sleep Cycle

Every ninety minutes you could fall asleep, given the right circumstances and motivation. Think of that after-lunch dreamy period, memorable to anyone who has worked in an office and had to endure boring afternoon meetings. The cycle is often recognized by a yawn. If you had to sleep in the afternoon before a night flight, note the time of that yawn. Add an hour and a half and modify your life. By that time, in fact ten minutes before it, be in bed in a darkened room. Make sure you have everything done, maybe read a book (airline manuals are great for this) with a light shining onto the white page and reflecting into your eyes. As the ninetieth minute approaches, a wave of tiredness will sweep over you. As soon as you notice it, close the book, turn out the light, and snuggle down to sleep.

Practice makes perfect and after a while you will be amazed how often this will work for you.

The Daily Poo

Getting in touch with your body's cycle can help you monitor and beat jet lag too. Listening to an expert on poo (a gastroenterologist) she said,

'It's simple: nine, nine and nine! You need to go once a day, it should be at 9 a.m., be nine inches long, and take nine seconds!'

Brown is good. Red, yellow, white and black are signs that something is amiss inside and you should see your doctor. There are differing consistencies, which can point to other facets of your health at the time. (As a result of the "The Black Poo Attack" our Mum discovered that we had been walking to school and spending our bus money on licorice blocks).

There are some very, repeat *very*, instructive websites that explain all this better than me[11]. I suggest you learn what healthy poo is and how to achieve it. Are you drinking enough water? Vegetables? Are you eating too much meat? Do you eat enough roughage? Monitoring your daily poo can give you a how-goes-it to see how your body is feeling.

Same with urine. Your urine should be the color of gin that is, clear, if you are hydrated properly. Clear to a light yellow in color is good. Anything bright yellow to orange shows you are not getting enough water. If you take supplementary vitamins, especially vitamin B, your urine will be brightly colored.

One doctor remarked that in his first year of medical school, he discovered the only thing taking vitamin supplements could do for you was to produce expensive pee and nothing had appeared to him in the thirty years since to change his mind[12]. He was referring to the words of a co-author of a study in the *Annals_of Internal Medicine*[13] who had completed a study of supplemental vitamins:

> 'What <u>will</u> protect you is if you spend that money on fruits, vegetables, nuts, beans, low fat dairy, things like that ...' then adding, '... exercising would probably be a better use of the money.'

The more in touch you are with your body, the more you can understand changes in your system. And use the signs to help you cope with changing sleep patterns. On layovers you will find that your daily constitutional bowel movement (who comes up with these names?) occurs at different local times. Flying to the other side of the world means that it's not unusual to have your "daily constitutional" *after* your local dinner before going to bed. It can be a little freaky.

When you go on holidays across the world a sign that you are beating jetlag is the change in your daily constitutional as your body moves closer in time. Eventually you will be adjusted to your regular 9 a.m., after you have woken-up and broken your fast. This takes at least three or four days, sometimes as long as a week. So your friends who think you are super human because you regularly battle jetlag are incorrect. Your body is like everyone else's, just a machine.

Look after the machine and listen carefully to its operation. The more you are in touch with the machine the better you can sleep on demand.

RECAPPING:

- **Take notice of your body's sleep cycle and use it to your advantage.**

- **Monitor your health by observing your daily excretions.**

- **Understand that you can't beat jetlag, just observe and plan for it.**

From the Logbook

If you live in the Middle East and your "daily constitutional" occurs at 9 a.m. local time and you find yourself, say, in Shanghai's Underground Market at 2 p.m. you can expect that you will soon need toilet paper. At 2:10pm that need becomes urgent, and important.

Good luck.

A (*hard learned*) travel tip: NEVER leave your hotel in China without taking a daily supply of toilet paper with you.

After reading this British photo-journalist, **Navjot Singh**[14], who spent 11 years working in China, added:

'In most parts of Asia, public toilets are not clean. Often there is no tissue paper, no flush, the toilet is just a hole in the ground rather than a seat, and there's no soap (even in paid toilets).'

He suggests visiting aircrew:

'... take the hand wash soap from your hotel bathroom, a bottle of water and pack of tissues. (in China, you get perfumed tissues that are smeared with anti-bacteria), PLUS a small bottle of anti-bacterial hand cream. Even shopping centers can't be trusted, head for a five star hotel if you need a toilet.'

Caffeine

Each person has their own physiological response to caffeine, nicotine, hypoxia, the amount of sleep they require and so on. At your age you should understand how coffee affects you. What you may not know is coffee takes about twenty minutes to have an effect and can keep you alert for up to seven hours. You will read in the NASA nap section of this book that aircrew often have a coffee before their twenty-six minute nap, knowing they can get the benefit of the nap before the caffeine kicks in.

If you are having sleep problems, ditch the coffee. And how do you do that, besides avoiding Starbucks, Costa or Tim Horton's? First you have to know where the caffeine is, before you can begin to avoid it. The Mayo Clinic's website[15] and Health.com[16] are good starting places for further research. For the purposes of this book, note that decaf coffee can contain up to 20% of the caffeine of a normal coffee.

Caffeine is found in such obscure locations as:

- Tea - black and even green tea
- Soft drinks
- Chocolate (dark chocolate has more)
- Coffee-flavored ice cream (even chocolate-flavored has a little)
- Diet pills

- Some pain medication
- Sports drinks
- Energy drinks
- Breath fresheners
- Energized Sunflower seeds
- Some instant oatmeal products
- Some beef jerky products

One coffee a day may be good for you, but make midday your limit if you want to sleep well. As shift workers, aircrew have to plan their rosters in advance, adjusting their caffeine intake to suit. Using coffee to give you a boost before landing, during a night flight, is a good use of its properties. Most crew use it too late, when they are already feeling tired, and suffer through the landing and then can't sleep when they get home. Try bringing your coffee hit forward, to a geographical point say, 600 nautical miles to landing, so the kick arrives before that head-nodding starts.

If you are lucky enough to have regular sleep patterns, regulated caffeine may not be a problem for you and you can take heart in the following. In June 2015 the Journal Of Clinical Nutrition reported that a Japanese study of 90,000 people over eighteen years found two to five cups of coffee a day may reduce your chance of dying from:

- Heart disease
- Cerebrovascular disease (stroke)
- Respiratory disease

The dietitian who reported the study on Melbourne radio said it wasn't about the caffeine level but about the 'coffee experience' as a whole. Better still, it did not matter if it was *posh coffee, instant or decaf.*

In my opinion, if you have a relaxed lifestyle that allows you time to stop for a coffee, then maybe you have the stress-free existence associated with a long life. If getting to sleep is an issue for you, then cut the caffeine.

RECAPPING:

- **Coffee works and can be used strategically to help during flights.**

- **It takes between fifteen to thirty minutes to work.**

- **It has a half-life of six hours, that is, after six hours 50% of the effect is still in you.**

- **It's in many obscure products.**

- **It is a diuretic and can lead to dehydration.**

- **It prevents you from sleeping, so in a normal day try not to have any in the afternoon and evening.**

- **A long term Japanese study found that two to five cups of coffee a day may reduce your chance of dying from heart disease, stroke or respiratory disease.**

From the Logbook

A wise Melbourne Doctor, Dr. Sidhu, once explained that he and his brother had done extensive tests as university students, when he was studying medicine and his brother law. They reckoned that every other second caffeine would spike the brain, keeping them alert. But during this spike any studied material, making new memories, would cease.

They were staying awake twice as long, but studying at 50% efficiency. They concluded that, faced with cramming for exams, it was best to get up early and go for a walk, reviewing in their minds the information studied the previous evening.

No caffeine at all, not even decaf tea.

Their quality of study, they decided, was much higher but they could only study for half the normal time before becoming sleepy. The more time spent sleeping was beneficial, allowing the subconscious to embed the lessons learned. He ended the discussion by suggesting that both he and his brother topped their classes.

Drugs - Illegal

What is it about life these days that make young people want to get out of their brains?

As kids when we wanted to escape reality we'd head off to the library and grab a free book. You could be transported from having to do the dishes, suffering under the lash of two older sisters who always made you dry, to a place where you are sitting behind Evan Green and John Bryson in their UDT World Cup Rally P76 approaching Tamanrasset in the Sahara Desert. If rain was lashing the windows you could soon be living in the Conshelf 2 habitat at the bottom of the Red Sea with Jacques Cousteau. On a hot night you could chill with Dr. Carpenter as his small band staggered towards Ice Station Zebra.

All information in the world is contained in books and, no matter how hard you try, you can never fill your brain. Just try. But taking a pill is easier than turning a page, even if that page turn is a swipe on a Kindle.

The mind-altering drugs, called '*Recreational Drugs*', are not made by American, German or Swiss pharmaceutical companies but instead by an unwashed spotty science student called *Brains* in a mobile home on bricks in a bushland hideout. He's striving to add one drop of tenderness, using a combination of chemicals found under the kitchen sink. *Yet another use for WD-40.*

There is no standardization or quality control. Why would people who are so paranoid about eating trans fats, genetically-modified grains, cage-laid eggs or processed pork, happily shove one of these drugs into their temple-like bodies?

The great thing about the airline industry is that we have twenty-four hour drug testing. It solves the problem of having to decide whether you are going to cross the line or not. With the decision taken out of your hands there is a good chance that you will never have to worry about this, but for those who do indulge: *it's not good for your sleep.*

If you do fall asleep there is a chance, like one 21 year old man from East Gippsland in Australia who smoked a poisoned batch of ice, you won't *ever* wake up.

Ice users develop sleep disorders. They stay awake for extended periods when effected by the drug and sleeping prolonged periods when coming-down from a high.

Cocaine users also develop sleep disorders. The drug causes fatigue but it also induces insomnia. An interesting aside: one successful cocaine treatment method involves psychotherapy along with *gambling.* By also stimulating the reward center of the brain, gambling can take the place of cocaine.

Heroin users have less sleep disorders compared to the two drugs above, but Methadone (one of the treatment drugs) causes sleep disorders. 40-60% of heroin addicts relapse.

RECAPPING:

- **Don't do non-pharmaceutical drugs.**
- **To expand your mind, read a book instead.**
- **Drugs don't lead to restful sleeping.**

From the Logbook

A colleague was married to a man who changed industries in his forties. The new career involved him attending a conference in Las Vegas. A few months later he started showing symptoms of stress and she smelled a rat when repossession men arrived at the front door to take away the car.

Things went downhill and it transpired that he had become addicted to Ice from just *one night* in Las Vegas. He covered his addiction well and used his deception skills to ensure his wife was none the wiser, while converting all their assets to cash. He even refinanced their family home without her knowledge. Their lives have been ruined by the drug which, an Australian rehabilitation expert explained on Radio Station 3AW, has the toughest habit to break:

'We are seeing only a 2% chance of recovery from ICE.'

A more optimistic view is from an Arizona rehabilitator[17](maybe because it's financially lucrative to sell success):

'It is the reality of substance abuse and addiction that 75% of people who attempt to quit experience a relapse, at some point.

Most recovering persons experience four relapses prior to long periods of abstinence. For the addicted, recovery is a lifelong process.'

Drugs - Legal

We live in an instant world. Last week I read an inspirational article about a book written by the lead singer of Kiss, Gene Simmons. Within minutes, walking down the street, he was reading me his story, *Me, Inc.*

Instant audiobooks, instant money, instant music, instant photography, instant food, instant information, instant answers. Instant everything. So why waste time preparing for sleep and taking a risk you'll toss and turn when you can pop a pill and be off in the land of nod? Well, because most people don't take them as prescribed for a start. That is, as small a dose as possible for as short a time as possible.

While a short dose is possible to get over the shock of a bereavement, for example, it's no option when you have a flying career spanning twenty or thirty years. Often people increase the dosage as the body gets used to the drug and its effectiveness drops. Cold turkey results in "rebound" and the resulting case of insomnia is worse than the original. The fact that the quality of sleep is unhealthy is bad enough, but the side effects can be debilitating, even deadly.

We all have stories of trying a sleeping pill and waking-up feeling as if a semi-trailer had driven over us. My worst reaction was with one tiny antihistamine pill, a non-prescription drug to help with hay fever. Fourteen hours later I flew from Perth to Melbourne and back again through the night (including landing the 727 freighter) as if dragging my brain through molasses.

Here's a list of the side effects associated with all different types of sleeping medications:

- Clumsiness
- Unsteadiness
- Dizziness
- Light-headedness
- Daytime drowsiness
- Headache
- Nausea
- Drugged feeling
- Dry mouth
- Constipation
- Diarrhea
- Painful erections
- Sexual dysfunction
- Jitteriness
- Sweating
- Insomnia
- Weight gain
- Upset stomach
- Excitement or anxiety
- Dry mouth
- Skin sensitivity to sunlight
- Incomplete urination
- Faintness upon standing
- Increased heart rate

Can you imagine paying money to achieve these states? Not that you, in your entire lifetime, will experience all these side effects but even one is one too many. And it could be worse. The popular selling drugs Stilnox[18], Zopiclone, and Zaleplon have all been associated with neurological and psychiatric effects such as: sleep walking, sleep driving, sleep eating and sleep sex.

Zolpidem is reportedly used as a date rape drug.

A petition to ban Zolpidem[19] (Stilnox is one), Zopiclone and all other non-benzodiazepine hypnotics for the treatment of insomnia and other sleep-related disorders lists their reported side effects:

- "Hallucinations,
- nightmares,
- daytime drowsiness and fogginess,
- serious short-term memory loss,
- severe depression,
- weight loss,
- fatigue,
- loss of concentration,
- nervousness,
- confusion,
- anxiety and panic attacks,
- altered personality,
- loss of sexual inhibitions,
- paranoia,
- delusions,
- loss of rational thought,
- blackouts,
- amnesia,
- de-personalization,
- addiction,
- self-mutilation,
- psychotic episodes, and
- criminal behavior."

It is my opinion that Australia is a country addicted to Stilnox. The population is only 23 million and 1.2

million packets were sold in a single year. They have seen a number of patients experiencing strong suicidal thoughts as well as several reports of attempted suicides, accidents occasioning death, and completed suicides.

One young man fell to his death from an apartment tower, apparently during a Stilnox sleepwalk; and a huge media outcry resulted after a successful thirty-year-old woman fell to her death off the approach to the Sydney Harbor Bridge. She had been prescribed Stilnox for eight months instead of the recommended four weeks, and had recently been switched to Imovane to treat her insomnia[20].

The chances of you suffering such a life-threatening reaction are probably zero, but why take the risk? You're not cramming for exams here; you are planning to be in this industry for a long time. Not only are drugs risky, you can't even have an after-work glass of wine. The instructions for Stilnox plainly declare:

"Do not take Stilnox if you have been drinking alcohol or you believe that you may have alcohol in your bloodstream."

Plus, they cost money which could be more wisely wasted on chocolate.

Stilnox also responsibly states:

"It is not recommended for use for more than 4 weeks at a time."

If you plan on your aviation career lasting longer than that, it's time to turn to something else.

The placebo effect of having a box of sleeping pills in your overnight bag is not to be dismissed. If you don't trust yourself, wrap the box in sticky tape to make it impossible to open. Knowing that an emergency sleeping pill is at hand can make you feel less stressed about getting to sleep. Just resist the urge to take one.

If you must try sleeping pills, check with your Aviation Medical Doctor to find which is acceptable and obtain a prescription. Keep a copy of the current prescription in your suitcase, and check in advance with the country of entry's website to make sure it is not a prohibited drug. As international aircrew you are required to be aware of these matters. For example, the popular Codral cold tablet in Australia is a prohibited substance in the United Arab Emirates, which means jail.

RECAPPING:

- **Sleeping pills are not a long term option for aircrew.**

- **Under strict medical advice sleeping pills should only be used for a week or two, not a career.**

- **Never drink alcohol and use sleeping pills.**

- **If you are flying internationally, it is your responsibility to find out if there are restrictions on pharmaceutical drugs.**

- **In most countries you must be able to present a copy of your prescription to authorities.**

From the Logbook

A friend and his wife were flying on a BA 777 from Singapore to London. They were in first class, dressed in their free pajamas, and both took Stilnox as sleeping aids. Hours into the flight my friend woke to feel his ears pressurizing. As a pilot, he knew that the aircraft was descending. Realizing that the flight was diverting he woke his wife and told her to get dressed. Their brains were foggy, so foggy that getting dressed took all their attention. The aircraft was diverting to Delhi with a bomb threat.

After touchdown the Captain taxied to the bomb location and the passengers were rushed off the aircraft to spend two hours standing in buses while the Indian security forces combed the aircraft for the bomb. They found nothing and the plane was soon on its way. The Stilnox-affected pair were struggling to remain lucid.

At Heathrow immigration they reached into their hand baggage to discover that their money, passports, cameras and phones had been stolen back in India, presumably by the security forces who searched the plane. An embarrassed group of thirty other passengers were also discovering that, they too, were without passports; on the wrong side of the immigration fence.

He maintains that the Stilnox had turned his brain to jelly. A career long-haul captain, he maintains that he wouldn't have deplaned without at least slipping his passport into his pocket if had he been in his right mind.

If you cannot guarantee that you won't have to be roused from your sleep, due to fire, bomb-threat or other emergency don't take sleeping medication. Which means that it's worth learning the tricks to sleep naturally.

Fitness

There comes a time in your life when you start to value health. Probably in your forties. They say life begins at forty, not because you discover its meaning, but it's when you see death up close for the first time. It's usually the decade in which one of your parents dies. Nothing makes you grow up faster than turning off the life-support equipment and choosing a coffin. Nothing.

From being the carefree youngster, getting away with burning the candle at both ends, it coincides with a change in your metabolism. Those jam donuts and cakes start hanging around. Your uniform starts getting tight. At security they take longer when checking your I.D card, *'Yes, it's me!'* The hangovers last longer and take on a different edge.

If you're lucky, when you are in your thirties, one of your older friends has a mid-life crisis and you can observe the changes. A divorce, the appearance of the red car and, shortly afterwards, the twenty something-girlfriend. Within weeks, the gym membership appears and soon after, the juice machine arrives. The word *'wheatgrass'* enters your consciousness. Before long, lycra clothing and expensive white footwear herald the arrival of the bicycle. Not any bicycle, but one befitting an aviator: carbon fiber, with stupid pedals that require expensive shoes.

This gives way to the first broken wrist, a legacy of learning the hard way that the pedals must be unclipped when approaching a stop light. Only one thing in the world looks funnier than grown men drowning their cars at the local boat ramp every Saturday; it's the lycra-clad Michelin Man trying to stay upright on *the fastest bicycle on the planet* at the stop lights as he tries to extract his foot from the pedal.

If this is happening to your friend, heed the warning. In my case I was lucky that I was given the big brother talk (I don't have brothers), by one of my first airline Captains. He has remained a mentor and close friend until this day. *(Well, that was until he read this.)* He told me, and I am telling you: you ARE getting older and you MUST start getting fit. Best to make it a daily habit, rather than panic about vigorous gym sessions three times a week, because you are going to have to do this every day for the rest of your life.

In all baby-boomer suburbs, like something out of *The Living Dead*, every morning hundreds of men open their front doors and start walking the streets for forty-five minutes. Often within minutes of each other. In my Mum's suburb it was like wife-swapping pass-the-parcel. It was easy to imagine them all changing houses. But it wasn't that at all.

It was the heart attack sufferers. When you leave the hospital after being exposed to legal narcotics, seeing the face of god, and some hot nurses, the last thing your surgeon says is: *'You must walk forty-five minutes every day for the rest of your life'*.

Me, I am lazy. So I do thirty minutes a day now, in the hope that it'll stave off the heart attack. In the long run I hope to save fifteen minutes a day.

What sort of exercise?

Who cares? I reckon everything except running. It's my firm belief that we were designed to run short distances only when being pursued by sabre tooth tigers. And you can thank your forefathers and mothers that they achieved this important milestone. If you work out the physics of plonking your entire bodyweight on your foot, the stresses through your hips, knees and feet must be massive. And we all know runners who have had knee replacements in later life. Worse, we all know runners who has torn their Archilles tendon, or knee and they are out of the game for ages.

Remember, you have to do thirty minutes a day. Six weeks off isn't playing the game. And we all know how slowly the recovery is for those coming back from injury. Thirty minutes a day doesn't mean playing ball with your mates, where most of the time you are immobile before hamstring-busting spurts, then retiring to the bar to celebrate. That's a social activity. Thirty minutes a day means thirty minutes brisk walking, or riding, or jogging, or swimming. Something that gets your heart rate up. You know you're at the right level because talking should be getting difficult; especially if you are swimming.

As for gym work, and rotating each successive day, it's easier to do a few yoga classes and learn some effective stretches, then learn a few exercises to do using your own body weight. That way you can do your routine in hotel rooms before going for your walk.

A word about the "Athletes High". I have asked athletes about it. I thought it was as elusive as the G spot.

[On which subject Ben Elton pronounced, '*The best invention for women's sexuality was when they put toilet paper in those metal holders that you have to stick your finger in to start the paper off*.]

"Athletes High" is not some mind orgasm that occurs after you smash through an invisible wall of sound. It's a buzz you get *afterwards*, often in the locker room. For me it's the relief you'd get if you stopped banging your head against a particularly hard tree. And yes, it's OK; if you grew up before the 1960s.

Doing fitness makes you feel better, resulting in better problem-solving and a clearing of the head. You also get this smug grin, which is often mistaken for a grimace and the prelude to a heart attack. Your eyes will be brighter and soon you will like what you see in the mirror. Those of us who hate it with a passion (who wants to grow up anyway?) have discovered it's best done first thing in the morning.

Earbuds and a thirty minute current affairs radio program, podcast or audiobook make time fly. Music's OK, but people tend to have it up too loud and get run over, defeating the long-life benefits of the program. Anyway, time spent in hospital is time out of the game.

If you are a sad case (or it's wet, cold, and dark) try putting all your athletic clothes, socks and shoes right beside your bed. Chances are you can be half way around your block before you completely wake up. With the benefit of one of those mid-life sufferers as your mentor, encourage them to be your walking / cycling / jogging partner. They'll be waiting outside your door doing their 5BX Royal Canadian Air Force exercises[21] while you get ready. Better still, in a loud voice, they will give you fitness and dietary advice all the way along. All you have to do is grunt every few minutes. Afterwards you can retire to a cafe and treat yourself to huge cooked breakfast as a reward.

As with cancer cures, the internet is full of contradictory advice. You can find heaps of studies saying it's best NOT to do an exercise for four hours before you sleep. Others say you should flop into bed after completing a marathon every night. If you have to sleep during the day prior to a night duty it will come much easier if you have done some exercise during the day.

Have a look at:

The Royal Canadian Air Force 5BX system

It works. The comedian George Burns swore by it and lived to 100. Critics now say that you could injure yourself doing the sit-ups, so see your doctor before commencing an exercise program if your idea of exercise is fumbling under the cushion for the TV remote control.

Yoga Stretches

Make sure a professional shows you the correct way in order to gain the full benefit.

Simple Weight Bearing Exercises

Using only your bodyweight and no equipment. OK, the variable resistance rubber bands are excellent, and fit in your suitcase. Get proper training from a health professional first, preferably a physiotherapist.

Walking

Get good footwear and comfortable clothing. If you are using a treadmill, a tip passed on from one of my trainers was that the gradient should be no more than two units LESS than the speed in kph. Therefore, if you are doing a six kph (3.72 mph) walk, then the gradient should be no more than four degrees. If you have lower back pain, you should only walk on the flat.

Cycling

You don't have to attire yourself in the clothing of the latest Tour de France winner or own a carbon fiber bike to achieve the benefits from cycling. In fact, a heavy old clunky bike is better. You'll burn more calories getting it around the same distance and few people would want to steal it.

If you are new to the mode of travel, you need to get help before you begin. Technique is important. Safety plays a large part in your enjoyment of the activity. If you don't feel safe, you won't do it every day. Plus, you have a greater chance of being killed or injured on a bike than by walking.

You need a reliable bike, reflectors and lights, a bell, glasses (few things are as thought-concentrating as having a bug hit your eye when you're riding fast), bike helmet, bike gloves (to protect the flesh on your palms if you take a tumble) and a mobile phone. The phone is to call a taxi to take you and the bike to the bike shop if you get a flat tire. Changing or repairing tubes by the side of the road is for children and enthusiasts.

Cyclists sprout that *"Studies have shown that regular cyclists enjoy the general health of someone 10 years younger;"* although the studies must have been in secret because I cannot find them. Having cycled regularly for more than twenty years I can attest that my sister, the doctor, reckons my legs look good.

It's true that cycling is low impact which has to be better on your hips knees and ankles than running. It improves balance and co-ordination. Once on layover in Dusseldorf I was astounded to see ladies in their late seventies and eighties cycling to the shops. It has to be a factor in staying young.

Swimming

Like cycling, your proximity to equipment determines whether you'll be able to include swimming into your regular lifestyle. You don't have to spend much on the uniform, but you can't hide a pool on the balcony in the way you can hide your bike.

The benefits are enormous, as there is no weight-bearing involved, which is why aqua aerobics is used so widely for elderly arthritis sufferers, and for sportspeople recovering from injuries. Again, you have to make sure you are doing it right, or your face is under the water for longer than is life-sustaining. Calorie consumption is about the same as cycling. Nothing says that you can't mix and match your fitness to suit your lifestyle. Ten minutes on the exercise bike and twenty minutes on the treadmill adds a weight-bearing component, necessary as we age.

After exercise, you can add ten minutes of floating on your back in a pool, toes holding onto the edge while you meditate. Don't knock it, the astronauts had to fly to space to get a similar weightless experience. It can also get your daily Vitamin D dosage directly from the sun.

Most airlines have "crew clubs" with exercise equipment stashed in the all the hotels in their network. Mountain bikes in Munich and tennis rackets in Tokyo. For me, though, a layover is a treat. No gym, maybe a swim, but more likely walk, walk and walk. In a twenty-eight hour layover I can walk about two hours and take a few photos.

You need 150 minutes of exercise a week, twenty-two minutes a day. Or thirty minutes five days a week. Recent studies suggest you don't need to take the exercise in one hit. Ten minutes in the morning, ten at lunch, and ten in the evening puts you way above the national average, and soon shows benefits, leading to a reduction in the chance of:

- stroke
- heart attack
- diabetes
- osteoporosis and fractures
- obesity
- dementia (memory loss)
- depression
- high blood pressure
- colon and breast cancers

But most of all, exercise leads to better sleep.

RECAPPING:

- As you age, your health starts assuming a greater importance.

- If you are lucky you can use an older friend as a mentor.

- Your goal is thirty minutes of 'movement' every day: walking, jogging, running, biking or swimming.

- Stretches and some weight bearing exercises help too.

- Your weekly social sporting event doesn't count for much, the drinks in the bar afterwards negates the benefit.

- See your doctor and make sure you are up to it, if exercise is foreign to you.

- Get a referral to a physiotherapist who will teach you a set of regular exercises you can live with.

- A gym membership can be helpful if you live in a place with regular inclement weather, or can benefit from the camaraderie of other members and help from instructors.

- Obtain good footwear / equipment and learn how to use it correctly.

- Regular exercise leads to better sleep.

iPods, Audiobooks & Apps

How did we live without them?

It was a month after the Twin Towers fell that the first iPod emerged on the streets of New York. The concept of people listening to their own music as they walked to work made television news worldwide. This city was already distinctive for people who walked to work in business attire wearing Nikes. Whoever took two pairs of shoes to work each day? New Yorkers did. And now they had white wires hanging from their ears to go with their white shoes.

Rich people paying $339 ($600 in today's money) to listen to their own music rather than the city's excellent FM radio stations. Surely they'd run out of stupid, rich people before long. A few years later we could afford USB-sized MP3 players to replace our bulky cassette and CD players. My first one cost $30 and stored about twenty songs.

By 2004 iTunes was up and running, they'd sold their two millionth iPod and the iPod Mini had arrived. It was time to drink the Apple-flavored Kool Aid. Soon after I opened an account with Audible.com[22] my life changed for the better. Living in noisy Ho Chi Minh City in Vietnam, I could plug in my earbuds and select anything, from music, to a soundscape of my native Australia and audiobooks. The never-ending hum of the four stroke motorcycles that clouded the air vanished. My life improved. Yours can too.

Being able to control what you hear allows you to control your surroundings. Controlling your surroundings allows you to sleep when you want. You can get an iPod on eBay or buy them online brand new from Apple. I always have two: an iPod Touch and an iPod Nano, as well an app on my phone that allows me to listen to audiobooks. But phones chew up battery life, and I have a special use for them when I am sleeping as you shall see. Download the free iTunes program on your computer which, after you install it, will search your computer for every song you own. It also has an online shop from which you can purchase millions of songs and tracks.

Synchronize your iPod to your iTunes, and pair the two individual items. You choose what, of all your stored music, you wish to have on the iPod. iTunes allows you to make "playlists" of songs you want to hear. So rather than thousands of songs you can make a playlist of, say, your top 400, and only transfer those across to your iPod. You can also synchronize "podcasts" which are stored radio shows from radio stations and, more recently, programs made for the internet. iTunes allows you to find and "subscribe" to the podcasts, automatically obtaining the latest version and downloading-it to your computer.

You can spend hours surfing the internet sites of the British Broadcasting Corporation (BBC), Australian Broadcasting Corporation (ABC), and legendary National Public Radio (NPR) broadcasting system of the United States. The world's most popular podcast is "This American Life" produced by Chicago Public Media, including their offshoots "Serial" and "Planet Money." Another American classic is Garrison Keilor's weekly "The News from Lake Wobegon." The selections you have chosen for synchronizing your iPod to your computer can allow you to have all episodes of the podcasts on your iPod, the most recent, or only a few.

As well as songs and podcasts, iPods can hold video, photographs, TV shows, and books (although you have to have good eyesight to read on iPod-sized screens).

Where they come into their own is with audiobooks.

Everyone I have mentioned audiobooks to has countered: *'I could NEVER listen to an audiobook ...'* and proceeded to berate me for suggesting it. To them I say, *'Fine. Have a nice day.'* I am sick of trying to convince people, receiving massive pushback, and three months later being rung up in the middle of the night to be told that:

> *'Audiobooks are the best thing ever ... OMG! They are amazing, incredible, changed my life, etc. etc..'*

I know. It happened to me in my house in Saigon and I had no-one to ring. When it is right for you, go to audible.com and sign-up. You get a book for free and you can cancel your subscription anytime. They are now owned by Amazon, so you are probably already a member.

To kick-off, you are looking for one of four books to give you a welcoming introduction to the format:

In A Sunburnt Country
By Bill Bryson
(Called *Downunder* in Australia)

The Memory of Running
By Ron McLarty

The Power of One
By Bryce Courtenay and
narrated by Humphrey Bower

The Girl with the Dragon Tattoo:
The Millennium Trilogy
By Stieg Larsson and narrated by Simon Vance.

It's important you choose one of these four, and you must never get an *abridged* audiobook, unless it is a Bill Bryson book and he abridges it and reads it himself. You must hear them as the author intended and not how some young caffeine-addicted editor in a publishing house figured it should. Every word is there for a reason.

The narrator *makes* the audiobook experience, and often the writer who reads their own stuff knows when to pause for effect or how best to deliver an amusing line. Look for anything read by Simon Vance, Scott Brick, and Humphrey Bower. They have the ability to make various accents believable.

If the narrator is Bill Bryson, the famed travel writer, settle back and prepare to cry laughing as he recounts his travels around Australia (*In a Sunburnt Country*), the universe, your own body and everything in between (*A Short History of Nearly Everything*) or America's greatest summer (*America: One Summer 1927*). All his books are rare gems.

Having purchased your book, you will find it in Library / My Books on the Audible site. Always choose "enhanced audio or Number 4" for the quality level on the top right hand side. Then download the book to your computer. Once downloaded (you may have to look for it in your Downloads folder), double-clicking it should get it to play in your iTunes. Otherwise you can import it into your iTunes by selecting File / Add

To Library and locating the book in your Downloads folder. Now synchronize your iPod with your computer and iTunes, and choose to have your audiobooks appear on your iPod. If you use the Audible.com app, set up is even easier. See what is in your library and download whichever title you want to hear.

Clear the decks. Tell your friends you are going away for an hour or two; grab a cup of tea, find somewhere snug and press play. Shut your eyes and let yourself be carried away. If your mind wanders, rewind a few minutes and pick it back up again. And again and again, until you find yourself riveted to the spot. Like the first time you get meditation (if you ever have "got it"), you will float into a new world. Give me a concentrated hour of your time and I will have created another audiobook monster.

Besides novels, audiobooks are excellent ways of becoming educated in an entire range of non-fiction subjects: how to manage money, how to budget, how to invest in your future, becoming healthy, thousands of inspirational biographies, histories and so on. Name a subject and there are at least a few audiobooks on it. Test-listen to see if you like the narrator before you buy. Nothing is worse than a voice that grates. You can return a book that doesn't work for you and get a refund. The most economical way of becoming a member of audible.com is to put, say, $230 into your account and receive 24 credits, bringing the cost of a book down to under $10 each. Filling-up your iPod with a library of audiobooks means that you have one for every occasion.

There are also great audiobooks relating to meditation and sleep sounds. Guided meditation to help you to sleep, or you can use soundscapes to mask background noise and help you sleep better.

After failed attempts (recording rain has to be the second-most popular thing in the world besides sleeping), I found Matsushima Records who have produced "*Absolute Sleep Music - Rain Sounds for Sleep and Relaxation[23]*." It is available on iTunes, to be downloaded and made into a playlist.

iTunes is fiddly when it comes to making multiple copies of the one track in the same playlist. You have to copy the sound and then make another playlist. Copy all within it and paste it back into the original playlist. Repeat back and forth until you have about sixteen versions of the seventy-eight minute track. Now when you press play it will go for about twenty hours without stopping - a great mask for background noise; *make sure you empty your bladder before going to bed.* There is an option to repeat the 'song' but making a lengthy playlist means you don't have to keep changing settings every time you wake up. The aim is to have an iPod that is armed with listening pleasure no matter your mood. You'll be amazed how quickly your mood changes. What was a great idea when you were in line at the supermarket is not palatable at all when you are trying to sleep a few hours later.

The excellent novels and non-fiction books keep you entertained for hours while you are doing mind-numbing exercise to help keep healthy and lose weight. Losing weight helps you sleep better, being fitter helps you sleep better because your body needs sleep after exercise. In situations where you cannot sleep easily, listening to an audiobook while lying in bed in the dark helps you to sleep as it stops your mind racing with your own thoughts and the droning voice, at the right level, helps put you to sleep. If nothing else, it rests your eyes.

Always make sure that you set up an alarm within your iPod if there is a requirement to wake up. I use a loud song from within a special playlist that I have made rather than the iPod's beeping sound. As I always have other alarms, it is preferable to wake to a favorite song before all the noisy alarms go off. When you wake up after sleeping, wind back the podcast or audiobook to a point that you remember. No drama. By using audiobooks, podcasts, and soundscapes, we are going some way towards controlling your audio environment and part way to controlling your sleep.

Sleep Applications for iPad, iPhone and Other Phones

At the time of writing there are 490 apps in the iTunes store teaching you how to sleep. Everyone who made "sleep music" in the 2000s has got themselves an app developer. Having looked at a few of them I baulk at being told how to sleep by anyone. The idea is to learn the tricks to aid sleeping, try them out, find ones that suit you and apply them. That said, if you find an app that fits with your body clock, go ahead. Like the ideal hotel pillow and duvet combination, it's elusive for most of us.

Technical stuff you should know

Flash

Originally the iPod came with a tiny hard drive, which sometimes failed if dropped. These were superseded by the more robust flash drives that have no moving parts. If given a chance, buy one that uses flash drive technology.

Alarm

Some models of iPod (specifically the latest "Nano" and "Touch") come with a clock and alarm feature. You need this type. Check first. If you cannot set an alarm, give it a miss and try the next model. Always set an alarm if you are using the iPod for sleep purposes.

Earbuds

The iPod comes with a white set of earbuds. They seem to fit most people; but not me. I prefer the smaller in-ear Sennheiser buds, as I sleep on my side and these are more comfortable. The latest craze of wearing full studio style earphones, notably by Dr. Dre, may be excellent for walking around the street, but are not comfortable when you are curled up in bed. At press time, a new product was released: *Sleep Phones.* They incorporate headphones into a headband, and should be worth a look[24].

Bluetooth

Bluetooth headphones can work with the latest iPod Touch and Nano. Good for walking around the streets and in the gym, Bluetooth earbuds and headsets have no wires connecting the device to the earphones, but they are still a little bulky for sleeping. You can Bluetooth your iPod to your car's sound system, which is great for long distance driving while listening to an audiobook.

Caution

If you have been riding bicycles since you were a kid and already have a preoccupation mindset that everyone is out to kill you (*only the paranoid survive*), then walking around with ear buds jammed into your ears will not prove a problem for you. However, if your visual scanning is not highly-developed it can be dangerous to play loud music as you are walking. One of the benefits of podcasts and audiobooks is that the spoken word doesn't seem to mask street sounds as much. There have been quite a few deaths of people crossing railway lines, or crossing roads, while listening to iPods. If you don't have common sense, be extra cautious when out and about.

RECAPPING:

- **Get an iPod or two.**
- **Download and setup iTunes and an account.**
- **Subscribe to some free podcasts from BBC, ABC and NPR.**
- **Setup an account with audible.com.**
- **Buy some audiobooks.**
- *In A Sunburnt Country*
  - By Bill Bryson and narrated by the author.

    (Called *Downunder* in Australia)
- *The Girl with the Dragon Tattoo*
  - By Stieg Larsson and narrated by Simon Vance.
- **Set the alarm, in case you drift off.**
- **Give it a dedicated hour to listen to your first audiobook. If that title doesn't grab try another, and another.**
- **Have a look through the iTunes store for sleep apps. If one works for you, buy it and never lose it.**
- **Be serious about using an iPod while walking around. Lots of people, oblivious to their surroundings, have been killed by cars and trains** (*hopefully not at the same time*) **while listening to their iPods.**

Massage

Pure bliss is having a massage before you sleep. Ideally, in your own home, with a trained masseur who brings their own massage table. It's better if your massage therapist is *not* a friend so you can tell them when they are doing it wrong, or hurting you. When you are "helping" a friend who has done a massage course (and we've all got one), the chances are that you will get a discount but feel embarrassed about telling them what to do. This is important, because depending on the time and relationship to your flight, you want a different type of massage. If you are trying to relax before a sleep in the middle of the day prior to a night flight, you'll want a soft, calming massage.

If you have landed after fourteen hours jammed in a 777 cockpit seat you will feel as if you have been in a car crash and want a restorative massage. This may include muscle-kneading which, if observed, would have onlookers calling the police. A top massage therapist can read your body and, after you explain what you need, will modify the pressure appropriately.

Seek out someone who has recently become qualified, who has few clients and needs to gain experience. You want to do a trial massage. Based on a successful outcome negotiate to sign up for, say fifty massages at a reduced rate, with a free massage for every new person you introduce. That's one a week or so ordered and planned in advance after you get each month's roster. By building their massage timetable around your roster each month, the therapist can then plan their movements. Suggesting the days to their nearby customers allows them to pro-actively contact clients which is a win for them. At many destinations a massage can be much cheaper than at home and is the ideal reward for a hard flight.

In either case, beware of the 'sensual massage.' An untrained two-finger jab at your flab with the encouraging *'You like?'* is not a massage and can even result in bruising. After one "Swedish Massage" in Bangkok I was almost crippled for three days.

If a massage is not available, then a pre-sleep hot shower or bath can do wonders. Sadly, arriving exhausted at the hotel you promise yourself a hot shower, but inevitably crash instead.

RECAPPING:

- **Find yourself a masseur who you can direct as to the type of massage required.**

- **Consider a visiting massage service if you regularly do long haul night flights.**

- **Try to get a bulk deal and plan ahead every time you get a new roster.**

- **In many destinations where massages are cheap, the quality of the massages are dubious.**

From the Logbook

Leo, from China, spent years in university studying massage and has been running his own business for eight years. He has fingers like steel rods. You think you've had foot reflexology before, until Leo takes over. Then you realize how restorative it can be. He is a small man, strong and fit, who brings his own industrial-sized massage table to your home. Three of us use him regularly and he finds no need for confidentiality about his patients.

I am a softie and don't like the agonizing massages that leave you crippled for three days afterwards. But my two friends do. One remarked, during a massage,

'It must be exhausting for you to massage all day'
'Yes', he replied, *'Very hard, I can massage only ten hours a day.'*

He kept massaging, thinking, then considered:

'Except The Captain … it like massaging a baby. If all like The Captain I could work twelve, maybe fourteen hours straight.'

When you have an ongoing relationship with a top masseur don't try to do their job. One day I got back from a particularly long flight from Dakar, Senegal to the Middle East (a ten hour night flight) and figured I needed a neck and back massage.

Leo pretended to sympathize, and after the back and neck he was soon at work on my legs and feet as well. After experiencing the most-needed foot massage of my life I realized that you should leave it to the experts.

It is common to be hassled as you walk the streets of Hong Kong, Bangkok or even Shanghai by masseurs of dubious reputation. I have nothing against prostitution as a profession, but please don't pretend to offer exhausted air crew a massage then fail to deliver.

To such overtures a good response is:

'Happy ending?'

If this elicits a positive response you know it's not the type of massage you're after. Asking the following gets a confused glance and gives you time to make an escape:

'What about a happy beginning?'

Mosquitoes

In the last hundred years more American soldiers have become casualties of mosquitoes than bullets[25]. The females are the most dangerous living beings on the planet[26], killing 750,000 humans annually and destroying the lives of hundreds of thousands more[27].

Twenty years after returning from the war, U.S.Vietnam veterans who suffered:

- depression
- intense irritability
- severe forgetfulness
- had trouble sleeping

were found to be suffering from the after-effects of **Cerebral Malaria**[28] transmitted by mosquitoes. It had been passed off as Post Traumatic Stress Disorder (which they may have also suffered). After psychiatric testing, one had lost thirty I.Q. points compared with the test he'd taken before he went to war[29].

You don't have to be fighting in a jungle to have your life changed forever by a single mosquito; **Topaz Conway** just went to Malaysia. She told Australia's ABC Radio's Background Briefing[30]:

' ... *Suddenly felt like I was being attacked by an army of mosquitoes and I ran and they literally chased me back to my hut. So on day five when all the symptoms of salmonella went away, the pain came back and that's sort of when I lost the plot and told the doctor, 'You can cut off both my arms and legs because I just cannot live with this pain,' and I was dead serious at the time.'*

Her trouble wasn't Malaria but the new world-wide plague, **Chikungunya**[31], which was little known in 1990 and now infests sixty countries. As well as a hideous skin rash, the pain in your limbs becomes so great that you can neither hold your baby, wipe your bottom, nor open a fridge for weeks, months, or even years, even with maximum pain relief medication. You may even lose your sight[32]. And whereas the carrier of Malaria is a tiny mosquito, most active an hour before and after sunset and sunrise, Chikugunya gets around on the A380 of mosquitoes, the huge Asian Tiger mosquito. Not only active all day and all night, but it is aggressive as well. It even chases you.

Malaria kills 584,000 people a year, mainly kids in Africa. In the time it has taken you to read down this far since the chapter heading another one just died. And, in 29% of cases, they are the lucky ones, dying soon after being born. For the others, death comes after horrible suffering that drags out for years.

There is also:

- **Dengue Fever**[33], which the World Health Organization says affects 390 million people annually;
- **Ross River Fever**[34],
- **Murray Valley Encephalitis**[35],
- **Yellow Fever**[36], and
- **West Nile Virus**[37].
- **Zika Fever**

A cocktail of two of these, or a return bout o Dengue, can see you in hospital with Dengue Hemorrhagic Fever or Dengue Shock Syndrome. A nurse in Cairns, Australia told me during an outbreak:

' ... *we always have six patients where we just keep giving them blood transfusions. And it keeps pouring straight out ... from everywhere.'*

Follow the footnote links for more information if you want to become an expert, but you can take it from me that you do not want to afflicted by a mosquito-injected disease. It's not often that you read of diseases where there is *"no specific treatment and no vaccine,"* but that's how it is for all except Malaria which has the drug Malarone; and for Yellow Fever, which has an effective one-hit vaccine.

Like a car accident that leaves you in a wheelchair, your story immediately becomes two parts: *My Life Before Being Bitten* and *Now*. And, by the way, the ***now*** often lasts forever.

As one Vietnam vet put it[38]:

"Here it is 40 years later and I have an enlarged spleen, liver & kidney failure, anemia and a blood disorder."

The rest of your life is a long time to be crippled with medical issues. You can kiss goodbye to your aviation career and most of your hopes and dreams too. After one teeny, tiny, mosquito bite. Being aircrew, you most likely don't take precautions as you have heard the rumors about taking Malaria medication:

"OMG! :(It's bad for you!"

Be advised by someone who has done the research, the Malarone of today is a totally different drug to that used by your grandmother. It is safe and is constantly being upgraded. You can use it for 365 days in a row. So get over it, and get the drug. Take it exactly as prescribed.

Most malaria attacks are unobserved, since they happen in people's bedrooms away from reality television, so it's not often we discover what it's like. Here we can thank **Coumba Makalou** who has detailed her journey with the disease[39]:

'When I contracted malaria, an infectious tropical disease caused by parasites found in the female anopheles mosquitoes, I probably had the virus in my system for about three weeks before I realized I was sick. I just felt extreme fatigue, headaches, a complete loss of appetite, and fever. It just felt like the flu.'

'I realized I had contracted the disease, when the infection was already quite advanced in my blood and I suffered from a sudden attack in the middle of the night. I awoke to what felt like lightning going through my legs, and then spreading through my body and in my head. Probably the worst headache, body aches, and chills you could possibly imagine. It felt like I was being stung repeatedly by an electric shock gun and could barely control my movements. **The pain was so intense; I actually believed I was dying,** literally crying out in pain so bad that I was taken to a 24 hour clinic that night at 3am.'

'Because Malaria is as common in Mali as catching a cold in the US, the clinic was not panicked at all when I came in. The nurse saw me and said nonchalantly like it's the most normal thing:

"Oh, you just have malaria. You're lucky you came in because it can kill you".

They gave me tranquilizers for the tremors, anti-parasite injection and a blood test to confirm the diagnosis, and sent me home for the night.'

Her story is on the NothingButNets.net website, which challenges people to send ten dollars to buy a mosquito net which is the distributed by UNICEF, the United Nations or World Health Organization. (Who knows? You might save a life.)

Thankfully, men are so attuned to *Man Flu* that they call for help at the first sign of malaise. If I was as sick as Miss Makalou had been for three weeks there is a good chance that the United Nations would have already been advised, along with everyone I'd ever met. I'd have even taken out ads in the newspapers and started planning my funeral. But women are much more stoic, especially mothers who are juggling family responsibilities, and they may not seek medical help until it gets serious. Big mistake. You must tell your doctor that you have been in a dangerous area for Malaria (and other tropical diseases), even up to twelve months after returning home. As a profession they are clever, but can't be expected to know everything. Saying: *'I'm sick. Guess why!'* is not enough.

This book is about sleep, not blood-borne diseases, and my role is to teach you how to sleep in mosquito-affected areas. As a professional aircrew member you have to take responsibility for your own health. Ideally, you are working for an airline that employs at least one doctor who specializes in tropical and infectious diseases and ensures they go to the conferences to find out the latest information. Then tells their crew what to do.

If not, it's all up to you.

Determine the risk before your trip, see your doctor, get medication if possible; and get educated. The World Health Organization website is a good place to start. For everything except Yellow Fever and Malaria, there are no vaccines or magic pills. The medical profession puts you in a room and tries to keep you alive long enough for your body to beat the disease.

Even then, the death rate only drops from 20% to just under 3%.

It's that simple. One mosquito bite and you could die. Your brain could swell, you could have a stroke, or bleed from everywhere for weeks ... and then die. Or you could be in so much pain that you *want* to die. The Dengue mosquito is a day-time attacker, the Malarial prefers dusk 'til dawn. And, as I said, the Asian Tiger never stops.

So this is how to prevent mosquito bites[40]:

Shower

Be Clean. Don't use flowery scented perfume or aftershave.

Repellent

Use DEET personal mosquito repellent. The greasiest, slimiest, most uncomfortable mosquito repellent works. I find that it plugs the pores of my skin and makes for an uncomfortable evening so I only spray it on exposed areas: neck, arms and ankles.

Wash your hands after administering it, otherwise you will know about it when you rub your eyes. Bursting into tears over dinner is not confidence-building if tomorrow's passengers are staying at the hotel and they find out you are their captain.

Clothing

Use loose-fitting, long-sleeved clothing and long pants that are light in color (they are attracted to dark colors). Linen fabric is much lighter than denim; it does the trick and is not too hot in the tropics. Put on fresh socks and wear shoes rather than sandals.

Don't Drink Beer

They are attracted to beer and cheese so choose wine or spirits. The British Raj in India specified that you should drink gin and tonic, as the quinine in tonic water is an anti-malarial; but it is irrelevant these days as the quinine levels are almost non-existent.

Sit Next To Someone Who Attracts Them

We all have a friend or relative who gets devoured by mosquitoes, so sit next them. The flying vampires are also attracted to movement, so be still, and hope they fly right by. *This principle applies with sharks as well, but they only kill ten people a year.*

Sit in the Smoke

Most mosquitoes avoid smoke, maybe because it confuses their senses.

Sit in the Wind

They are not good at flying against strong winds, so will leave you alone if you choose to stand in a gale.

Stop Breathing

The real trick they have, which ensures their survival, is that they can sniff carbon dioxide from about thirty meters (thirty-three yards). While they can see you from ten meters (eleven yards) and feel your heat, it is the CO_2 you breathe out that attracts them. Since you can't hold your breath all night, it is best to prepare your room in such a way that you are alone when the lights go out.

Room Preparation

Upon arrival in a suspect location, check the room for fly screens, gaps around the windows, wall vents, and cracks under the doors. It's amazing what you can use to jam in these. Be inventive. Find a fun new use for toilet paper, the room service menu, stationery, and the dressing gown in the wardrobe.

After taking a shower, apply DEET and dress appropriately; cover the glasses and cups with tissues then douse the room with DEET room insect spray, turn on the air conditioner (inspect it to make sure there are no openings direct to the outside), and leave. Spraying lasts about two hours. After you return to your room it's a matter of not allowing visitors to join you. Often I find it more comfortable to wash off most of the DEET before sleep.

Mosquito Nets[41]

If you are with a dodgy airline and staying at a less than salubrious hotel, or are back-packing by yourself, a mosquito net is a must. There are many styles to choose from, the cotton ones are better than polyester and both of them breathe better than silk. Some nets are treated with *Permethrin* which is supposed to be a *"mosquito control product."* It lasts about two years.

Nothing, except the noise of firecrackers at midnight on New Year in China, prevents you sleeping as much as the sound of a female, pregnant mosquito who is hungry. Taking precautions against mosquitoes will help you sleep better. Guaranteed.

RECAPPING:

- **Female mosquitoes are the deadliest living thing on the planet.**
- **One tiny bite can give you life changing:**
  - **Malaria.**
  - **Yellow Fever.**
  - **Chikungunya.**
  - **Dengue Fever** (Dengue Hemorrhagic Fever or Dengue Shock Syndrome).

- o Ross River Fever.

- o Murray Valley Encephalitis.

- o West Nile Virus.

- o Zika Virus.

- Get vaccinated against Yellow Fever.

- Use Malarone prophylactic Malaria medication.

- Decide that you are not going to get bitten and take action.

- Get a mosquito net if there is a chance you will be staying in low-standard accommodation.

- Upon arrival in a mosquito-rich location:

  - o Shower regularly.

  - o Don't use strong perfumes or after shaves.

  - o Dress in light-colored, loose-fitting, long-sleeved shirts with long pants.

  - o Fresh socks (they love dirty ones) and shoes.

  - o Treat exposed areas of skin with DEET personal mosquito repellent.

  - o Wash the DEET off your hands with soap, in case you rub your eyes.

  - o Find gaps in your room and plug them up.

  - o Cover drinking utensils with tissues, then use DEET room spray in your room.

  - o Turn on the air conditioner and leave for a while.

- o Take your DEET personal repellent to dinner because members of your crew will not have brought any.

- o Stay off the beer and cheese, drink instead spirits or wine.

• Understand that some people attract mosquitoes more than others.

• Mosquitoes may avoid smoky and windy areas.

• If you feel unwell for up to twelve months after visiting a mosquito-rich area, immediately tell your doctor.

From the Logbook

There is a lady we know who delighted her family and friends by being a mosquito-magnet. One evening at a camp fire in a forest she noticed that mosquitoes were bypassing her and biting the man next to her. She seized the opportunity and ended up marrying him.

Highly-respected photographer **Michael Blamey**[42] contracted Cerebral Malaria while working in Vanuatu and experienced the same symptoms as Miss Makalou (above):

'For two weeks. Then I felt better. Got up, fell down, and went back to bed for another week'.

Asked to give you a personal message about embarking on a trip to a mosquito-affected area he suggested:

'Take something, use a net, cover up; you don't want to get bitten. Don't go. Choose another adventure.'

Dani Moger was living in Vietnam when she contracted Dengue Fever. She writes:

'Five days after being bitten by a mosquito at Ha Long Bay I started feeling unwell. A high fever came on very quickly (39.2 Degrees) and my body was aching. I went to bed. Quickly I became so weak I could neither get out of bed to get Panadol or call downstairs for help.

'Eventually I was well enough to get a Panadol and that helped. Rang the clinic and they asked me to come in but I was too sick to move. They suggested to stay comfortable and take lots of fluids until I could get there the next day.'

'Within 12 hours the fever was under control and the Panadol helped with the aches. Blood tests confirmed Dengue Fever, then each day the bloods were taken and levels checked to see if I need to be airlifted to Singapore'.

Having been a flight attendant for ten years, she knows your lifestyle and recommends:

'Maintain preventative measures. It's easy to get slack after travelling to affected places for a while without getting bitten. My case was mild. I have friends who turned black and blue from bruising. Dengue is a horrid disease. Maintain vigilance!'

Natural Remedies

The cockpit door has long been a separator of cultures. Inside are people who have made a huge financial, long-term career choice whose employment contract is renewed only by passing annual license and medical exams. Their ability to fly hangs on passing their medicals which are conducted by people whose total reliance is on scientific tests and approved pharmaceutical drugs. What they put in their bodies is regulated by legislation and approved by an army of "experts." By the time a pilot reaches an airline they have been brainwashed by the medical profession and had enough blood and samples taken to lay a CSI trail lasting decades. Tell a pilot you are about to take their blood and they'll make a fist and show you which vein is the best. For the duration of their employment, their annual hours allocation is "owned" by the airline. So they do what they are told.

Cabin crew, on the other hand, are normal people. Entry to the industry is much easier and less regulated. They only seek medical attention to get well, and may even know what the inside of a health food store looks like. They believe in natural remedies and are more likely to try them out. Two such remedies to aid sleep are Melatonin and Valerian. Neither are offered to pilots by their Aviation Medical Examiners. In fact, in the 1990s when Valerian first emerged, pilots in some countries were banned from taking it.

Melatonin

Deep inside your brain is the pineal gland. It's the closest thing to your body clock. At night, it secretes Melatonin which helps regulate your sleep. As we have seen, you sleep: *you live*. You don't sleep: *you die ... after going crazy beforehand.*

Supplemental Melatonin does not put you to sleep. It doesn't. And the chances of you being deficient in Melatonin are millions to one. Whose great idea was it to produce tablets of the stuff and con you to ingest them in a desire to trick your brain? Especially when we know more about the Moon, than we do about this super computer which reminds us to breathe every few seconds, and beats our hearts with exquisite timing 100,000 times every day. This memory device in your skull which will remember every book we have ever read and never fill up.

Great idea. Tell them to try it on someone else.

Yes, taking Melatonin can shift your sleep *cycle* (to the tune of only thirty minutes, compared to two hours by light therapy), but it won't help you sleep *better*. For healthy people it is only recommended for short term use, up to two months. And what do we know about air crew who find something they like? Like their favorite restaurant near the hotel in Osaka, they will use it to distraction. Which means that if you convince yourself that it works for you, you will soon find excuses to live on the stuff.

The side effects include dizziness, daytime sleepiness, headaches, vivid dreams and even nightmares.

Oh, and remember: you may not drink alcohol when taking Melatonin supplements.

To confuse things, the supplement is not the same type of Melatonin that your brain produces and since it is not a controlled drug, there is no quality control over the production process. Your brain's ideal dose is about one tenth to one fifth of what's in the pills. Even if it was the same type in your brain, you are overdosing by a factor of five to ten.

The Mayo Clinic's Dr. Brent Bauer[43] has turned his mind to the issue and points out on their website that other, but less common, side-effects of Melatonin include abdominal discomfort, mild anxiety, irritability, confusion and short-lasting feelings of depression. Worse, it may react with medications you may be taking for blood thinning, suppressing your immune system, for diabetes or for birth control. If you are considering taking Melatonin for sleeping, see your doctor first. Seriously. In fact, see a sleep doctor. Pay them money to talk you out of it. I point you to the Mayo Clinic's website and anything Dr. Bauer suggests. This is not to say that Melatonin treatment is not a wise idea for clinical use. It has some effective results in old, sick people.

Despite what we say in the crew room, working for airlines isn't a sickness, it's a career choice. You shouldn't embark on tricking the most important clock you'll ever need, just to earn a living. It says *"Do Not Operate Heavy Machinery"* on the label, and there are few heavier machines than airliners.

Valerian

The root of the Valerian flower is crushed and made into capsule form which people take for a short term (two weeks), to treat insomnia. The advice issued by Australia's CAA in the 1990s suggested that the amount taken to have an effect could result in brain damage. There is no clinical proof that Valerian works in the recommended dosages. As with Melatonin, there is no quality control as to the production of the capsules and some have been known to have contained other, less healthy, ingredients.

Some people have serious reactions to Valerian, with drugs.com[44] listing common side effects as:

- Blurred vision
- Changes in heartbeat
- Headache
- Morning grogginess
- Nausea

Severe side effects include allergic reactions such as:

- Rash
- Hives
- Itching
- Difficulty breathing
- Tightness in the chest
- Swelling of the mouth, face, lips, or tongue

It is worth reading the latest information from reliable sources such as Drugs.com or the Mayo Clinic[45] website before entertaining thoughts on using Valerian. You *must* see your doctor before taking it and, like Melatonin, you cannot drink alcohol while using it.

There are restrictions while taking Valerian, including not being allowed to operate heavy machinery. How heavy is heavy? Is driving your car to an airport OK, but piloting an Airbus A320 unacceptable? And for how long after taking a pill? Seven hours? A month? For victims who may put their flying license at risk it's too hard. There are too many unknowns. Better to modify your lifestyle to induce restful sleep if you are considering a career lasting longer than a fortnight.

Top rating Melbourne Breakfast radio host, 3AW's Ross Stevenson, regularly pronounces:

'No-one has ever changed their point of view as the result of an argument.'

Which is to say that when confronted by friends, relatives and herbalists who proclaim you should take this potentially license-busting drug, don't argue. We all know someone who swears by these and other methods, and if the placebo effect works for them, who are we to burst their bubble? Thank them for the advice, smile, and say that you will see if it is approved by your Aviation Medical Examiner. Until you retire (or get caught), it is the AME who determines what can be put into your body.

RECAPPING:

- Supplemental Melatonin supposedly tricks your pineal gland in your brain by dosing you with five times the amount the brain secretes.

- Melatonin does not put you to sleep; it can only shift your sleep cycle by up to thirty minutes.

- Both Melatonin and Valerian may only be used for two weeks, have side effects and can react badly with drugs you are taking.

- You must see a doctor before taking either Melatonin or Valerian.

- You cannot use alcohol while taking either.

- You may not operate machinery while using either, and an airplane is a machine.

- The production of natural remedy supplements is not regulated; there is no standard as to what they may contain.

- Don't try to change peoples' minds when they tell you how good their experience has been; rely on your Flight Medical Examiner's advice.

Nicotine

Smokers find it takes longer to get to sleep, their sleep is "shallower," not as sound, and that they sleep less. It is generally agreed that the nicotine, not the delivery system, is what affects your sleep. People chewing nicotine gum or using patches also report the same symptoms. Anyone who has been a serious smoker knows that pleasure of waking up, having a cigarette, and then going back to sleep. The body craves nicotine and even wakes you up to get it. Sadly, especially in winter, it leads to smoking in bed and fires. Don't even allow it. If you want a cigarette in the middle of the night, make it your routine to get out of bed and smoke "safely".

Not that smoking can be considered safe.

On average, smokers die at about seventy-five years of age, with a cancer that grows so rapidly in the end that they can't get enough air to breathe. In actual fact the oxygen level that can be recovered by the lungs is below sustainable, even with supplemental oxygen. Once it gets below ninety the nurses remove the oxygen mask as there is no longer a chance of recovery.

Slow motion hypoxia is what happens next with the patient feeling that an elephant has sat on their chest.

Trying to breathe takes all their attention. Caring medical staff administer morphine, so the patient floats off in a happy drug-fueled fog, and muscle-relaxants are given so the family doesn't have to witness the shaking associated with oxygen deprivation. It takes quite a few hours before life departs.

Giving up smoking may help you to achieve a happier exit, and give you a few more years on the planet. In a short time your lungs and skin will reward you for quitting, and the benefits for doing so can be found elsewhere.

During the quitting phase, you can expect some memorable dreams and broken sleep. Physically and financially, the drama of quitting is worth it. Remember that the nicotine is out of your blood, urine, and saliva within four days, (hair samples can detect its use up to ninety days), but it can be agreed that after five days your body is free of the drug. It comes out through your skin, so saunas and lots of showers initially can help you feel better. From then on, it's all in your mind: a mental battle between you and the faceless board of directors of your tobacco company who are betting that you are too gutless and weak to beat them.

Understand that they are using the best marketing brains and dirty tricks in the world to tip the odds in their favor. They are laughing at you, driving top of the range BMWs and putting their kids through expensive schools thanks to you. Learning to dislike them may help you win the psychological war.

The danger periods for a reformed smoker are:

- Three days
- Three weeks
- Three months
- Three years

These are times you let your guard down thinking that you have it licked. But you haven't. Like love, it takes three tries at giving up before you have the strength to resist.

Don't beat yourself up if you lapse. Try again. And again.

Worse, even after ten years off the smokes, sometimes you will have a weird dream that you have lapsed and have fallen off the wagon. You will dream the sorrowful feeling of being annoyed with yourself then wake to find, with relief, that the Board of Directors can go fish for another victim. The money you save is considerable. Work out how much you spend on cigarettes and make sure you keep up with inflation. If you save it to a holiday account you can have a free holiday on the Board of Directors every year for the rest of your life. Why not take a *"Big Tobacco Cruise"* every year?

RECAPPING:

- Smokers don't sleep as soundly as non-smokers.

- Nicotine is a difficult drug to beat, but the rewards are worth it.

- After five days of not smoking, the nicotine is out of your system.

- The rest of the withdrawal process is in your head.

- Get strength to quit by having others help you.

- Imagine a battle of wits between you and the board members of Big Tobacco who reckon you are weak.

- 3 days, 3 weeks, 3 months and 3 years are times when you let your guard down.

- It takes most people three attempts before they finally quit.

- Even after ten years, you cannot have one cigarette. Not ever.

From the Logbook

One drag, on one cigarette, is enough to get you back, hook line and sinker.

A television director we knew had not smoked for ten years. One day his team won a prestigious award for the best sporting broadcast in the country for the year. During the (very) boisterous celebrations he was offered, and smoked, a cigar. The next day he was back to three packets of cigarettes per day, as if he had never given up.

One doctor, who uses hypnotherapy to help patients quit, says:

'Give me a heroin addict any day! Nicotine is the most insidious drug on the planet. What hope has the addict got? You are up against some of the best advertising and marketing brains in the world! People who give up are real heroes.'

A life-changing moment for me was giving a friend a lift to an Alcoholics Anonymous meeting, and then, as I was parking the car, the challenge: *'Come inside, it doesn't take long'*. We sat in the back pew of an old church, the front pews had been replaced with old lounge chairs. The meeting was already in progress. A forty-ish slender man made his way to the lectern. He never looked up and declared in a small voice:

'I am John; I am an alcoholic.'

The quiet church thundered with heaps of people responding,

"Hi, John!"

On closer examination there were people everywhere, lounging on the floor below the lectern, standing next to a coffee pot against the wall; this wasn't like any church service I'd imagined. There were no flowers and it all looked a bit dusty. A shaft of sunlight focused on the pews making the rest of the place appear dark.

For the next five minutes John launched into a story of his downfall and how he managed to get and stay sober. It was jaw-dropping. Inspirational. When he said that he had been sober for twenty days there was a cheer and when he sat back in the audience everyone chimed:

'Thanks John!'

It was only then that his expression changed and he broke into a sheepish grin.

As person after person shared their experience, I realized I had stumbled upon a gold-mine of the most enthusiastic, toughest, most-focused, inspirational people of all time. Their staggering crashes, resurrections and daily struggles made my life seem shallow. The energy of their presence was palpable. These were survivors who had been knocked-flat and crawled back-up, again and again … and again. Some had seen their own death close-up and knew they were on their last chance.

There were people who would be sleeping under a bridge that night, and others who may have been business leaders or judges. First names only. My friend told me of the time a top Hollywood actor had stood up in this very place, he was making a film in Melbourne, and told his story:

'I am Tony, and I am an alcoholic[46]'.

This was before *The Silence Of the Lambs* and only a handful of people recognized him. None acted starstruck and all treated him as an equal.

Halfway through our meeting a young girl; maybe seventeen, maybe twenty-six; shuffled in and slid into the pew next to us. Her head was forward and hair fell over her face. I noticed her shoulders heaving and heard a sniffle. A few huge wet tear blotches hit the sunlit wooden floor. My friend reached out and held her hand, squeezed it for maybe ten seconds then let go again. The tears soon stopped but the head never came up.

About five minutes later she quickly left as if she had forgotten to feed a parking meter. And didn't return.

My friend later said:

They usually take three meetings before they will even lift their heads up. It might be months before they can share.

It was only then I realized how strong you had to be to beat the bottle. My drinking habits changed immediately. I've never had a drink by myself since.

I turned back to the speaker, this time a seasoned professional whose story was now a stand-up routine, she was concluding:

' *... I have been sober for 483 days!*'

She paused for applause and murmur of support then finished with:

But I am still on the **smokes** *... one thing at a time, my friends, one thing at a time,*" drawing the loudest cheer of the meeting.

Every alcoholic in the room knew how hard it is to beat nicotine.

Get Help To Stop Smoking (or Drinking):

- United States of America ([47]&[48])
- UK[49]
- Australia [50]
- You can hear **Tony,H.** giving a talk about quitting drinking[51]
- You can hear **Buzz, A.** giving a talk about quitting smoking and drinking[52].

Rosters & Diaries

Getting control of your roster may be the biggest thing towards a better life, and better sleep. Having been in the business for thirty years I can confidently say that, after 360 monthly roster periods, I know three things about rosters:

1) Rosterers hate all air crew
2) If you bid for something you won't get it.
3) If you never expect anything, you'll never be
   disappointed.

Aircrew have to "bid" for the work they want to do in the following month. This includes what days they would like off, the individual flights, the types of flights, the destinations, either fly-thru or layover, as well as combinations of hours off. In some airlines you can bid to fly with (or avoid) certain staff numbers (although my friend tells me that if you try to bid to fly with your wife it *never* works).

It's a lottery. Every month it's like getting a Christmas present, except your present is often less than desired and you can't return it. The trick is to invest some time learning the system so that you understand how roster bidding works in your airline. Get help from healthy, happy people who seem to have a pleasant disposition. They seem to have the roster system working for them.

Do not spend a minute listening to someone who is a complainer, whiner, or who has dark circles around their eyes. They are obviously being overrun by the system, which means that they haven't mastered the tricks.

Plan ahead

Look at your next month, capture future events, holidays, birthdays, functions way out in advance. Spend a few hours planning your next month. Be realistic. If it's a rotating roster, you know that life down the bottom is going to be horrible. On those months only bid important days off, and don't expect to get them. Often, for evening birthday parties, it is prudent to bid for no flying after, say, 3pm one day, and none before midday the next. This allows full flexibility; you are still doing work and getting the time off you want.

Determine what type of work you want. Are you a morning person? Plan your roster around how you prefer to sleep.

Get help from more experienced staff members. Contact the roster team (despite the fact that they hate all of us); often they will happily give you bidding tips. When you make your bid, save it. Make a screen shot and keep a copy. Close out of the system, then login again and see if your bid is still there, saved as you wanted. Then save it again. Remember, we are dealing with billions of zeros and ones here; if something can go wrong, it will.

Roster Day

When the roster comes out, set aside two hours (while listening to an audiobook / podcast) and plot all your work into a calendar. Then print it out and have it on hand. Better still, see what the inspirational **Angelia Trinidad** has produced with her *"Passion Planner.53"* With nifty colors you can block off personal time, work, and sleep, capture your To Dos and do some creative mind-mapping at the same time. After more than fifteen years of struggling with electronic diaries on organizers, computers, phones, and iPads I have come to the conclusion that pen and paper suit me best.

When you are talking with friends don't agree to anything UNTIL you have checked your roster. Smile but say 'No!' :

'I'd love to BUT I will probably be working,
let me get back to you.'

And then promptly get back to them. Be a planner and a completer. Don't be an *'I'll be there if I can ...'* and then not RSVP or turn up. That works for a while, then you stop getting invited.

Just because you are an aircrew doesn't mean your life is more important than your non-shift working friends. Get a reputation for agreeing to turn-up at events, on time. Few other people are there on time. You can have a meaningful chat with your host without being interrupted, and slink off early if necessary. No matter how you try to explain it, your non-shift working friends and family will never understand your ways. That's OK; they have never seen the sunrise from a flight deck at 35,000 feet and can't understand that to be there to see it you have to get up at 2 a.m.

As you plan your calendar, also plan your sleep. Block out eight hours of sleep before every duty. The first month when you arrive at work fresh for every duty will be memorable. The flights will go faster, you will be happier, and you will feel in control of your life. It's addictive. You will feel that you have achieved much more outside of your work than before.

Do it three months in a row and it'll become a habit.

RECAPPING:

- If you never expect anything, you'll never be disappointed. Put in your bid, but remind yourself that the world isn't going to end if you don't get what you want.

- Investigate everything you can about your airline's Bidding System. Read the manual. Get help from the rosterers or from other crew who appear to be working the system.

- Take time to plan your "ideal" next month and bid accordingly.

- If yours is a five or six month rotating system, be real: only bid for important days off in the bottom months.

- When the roster comes out, take two hours to plan the following month, blocking out eight hours of sleep before duties, including preparation and travel time.

- Be tough on yourself to stick to your plan.

- RSVP to invitations and force yourself to be where you say you'll be, and be on time.

- The result is to feel that you are in control of your life, you'll keep friends and family happy.

- You will end up sleeping better.

From the Logbook

RVSP - Depending on your age, you may not understand this old-fashioned French concept: *"Répondez s'il vous plaît"* (Respond, if you please). There's a chance your grandmother may even be too young know of it. At the bottom of a written invitation these four letters alerted the recipient that they had to give the host an idea of who would be attending by a deadline date.

These days everyone is always hoping a better offer may come along, so they give some half-hearted excuse, then ring up at the exact moment all the guests are arriving and spend five minutes relating some lengthy story explaining why they aren't there. Invariably they end by asking, *'So what's happening in your life?'* as the stressed host cradles the phone while hanging coats, pouring drinks and mouthing *'Hello'* to those who have bothered turning up.

If you have ever seen the sad face of someone who has put on a huge party for thirty, including providing food and drinks, only to have six people turn-up then you will know how rude it is not to RSVP, or say you'll come and then fail to keep your promise.

The famous sales master, Zig Ziglar, used to say that there are only three types of people:

- Those who make things happen
- Others who watch what happen
- And those who say: *'What happened?'*

Getting control of your life by *making things happen* is the difference between loving this career or being chewed-up and spat-out by it. Your roster is just as hideous as the next person, but your *perception* is that you are controlling it, by planning ahead, with a subsequent rise in satisfaction. Formula one car racing and Australian football are important to me. By bidding for *time* off, rather than *days* off, I have been able to see nearly every event I have desired for the last four or five years.

Recently, after flying to India and back all night, I slept for two hours and then came out to my apartment's communal swimming pool to get some sun and drink my mug of tea. Sitting on the sun lounge next to me was one of the legends, a retiree named **Karim** who is there every day. As long as his tenants in Lebanon and London pay their rent he is a happy man.

It was during this conversation that I was reminded of family and friends who don't understand shift work.

After I explained I had been flying all night he said:

'Do you have to work today?'

I was incredulous:

'What are you talking about? I have been flying all night!'

'Yes, but do you have the rest of the day off?'

'Yes, I do'

He was happy for me:

'That's great then! A day off!'

I gave up trying to explain that flying all night was actually work.

"If you think that adventure is dangerous,
try routine - it's deadly!"

- Map Researcher, Daniele Quercia, **or**
  Author Paulo Coelho

Snoring

Snoring can result in a less than ideal sleep experience for the snorer: waking up with a sore throat, sometimes irritable, and feeling tired throughout day. For their partner, though, or anyone within earshot, it can mean that quality sleep is impossible to obtain.

What causes it? And what can be done to stop it, allowing all parties to get a good nights' sleep? There are two issues here, normal snoring[54] and sleep apnea. Snoring annoys you (and your partner[55]), sleep apnea can kill you and will be dealt with in the next chapter. Snoring is caused by air going in and out of the throat vibrating the soft palate and/or uvula.

The following factors can lead to snoring[56]:

- Being overtired.
- Being male. About 40% of men snore and only 25% of women. Up to 10% of children snore every night.
- Pregnancy. (In women, silly. Getting your wife pregnant is not enough to start you snoring).
- Putting on weight, especially around the neck. Those with a body mass index (BMI) over 30 particularly. To calculate your BMI

get yourself a free app, search the internet for a tool that performs the calculation for you or click here[57].

- Smoking, as it affects your airways.
- Drinking alcohol, especially in the last four hours before sleep. It even makes non-snorers snore.
- Taking medication that results in muscle relaxation, tranquillizers for example.
- Getting older. As my friend, a urologist, explained, *'Really, humans are meant to be dead by forty.'* Without exercise, as you age things start wearing-out, going soft and flabby. After fifty, snoring increases in both sexes.
- Having the wrong parents. Genetically narrow airways also cause snoring. (A lively discussion point at the next family dinner).
- Suffering a cold, allergy or nasal-blocking illness. Some people only snore when their mouth is open and they are not breathing through their nose.

When combined with sleeping on your back, conditions are ripe for producing a sound that is only rivaled by horny male koalas looking for a mate. If you have ever been lucky enough to sleep in a tent when one wanders past, twanging the guy ropes, as he serenades; you'll know how loud that can be. Otherwise follow this link[58].

In all the research reviewed there is no mention of *why* we snore. Maybe it helped our caveman forefathers from being eaten by monsters when they slept. Put yourself in the paws of a hungry mountain lion standing at the entrance of a cave filled with snoring humans. The din may have put our solitary koala to shame. Come to think of it, maybe the koala, upon hearing humans snoring, came to investigate the female talent.

What if you live alone and have no complaints? Here technology comes to the fore, get your hands on a voice activated recorder app, and record your sleeping. Having discovered that you snore, fixes[59] are simple:

- Change bedrooms or get single.
- Lose weight.
- Take up exercise.
- Stop smoking.
- Don't drink alcohol in the four hours before bed, or cut out the types that cause you to snore (creamy liqueurs, red wines and port are often the culprits).
- Change muscle-relaxant medication and knock-off tranquillizers.
- Don't sleep on your back. Sewing a tennis ball on the back of your pajamas is known to help.
- Sleeping in a chair, or propped-up with pillows and cushions may fix the problem.

If the snoring is loud, stops then resumes, sometimes causing you to wake up with shortness of breath, tired, with a headache, or you find yourself falling asleep during the day, then you may have *Sleep Apnea* which can cause your life to end much earlier than you'd think.

RECAPPING:

- If you are unaware if you snore, record yourself with a voice activated recording app.

- Is your snoring "normal" or Sleep Apnea?

- Lose weight.

- Stop smoking.

- Take up exercise.

- Don't drink alcohol for four hours before sleep.

- Try to avoid wines and liqueurs, and foods (like cream) that can set you off.

- Stop taking tranquillizers, see your doctor and change medications that make you snore.

- Sleep on your side, sew a tennis ball onto the back your pajama shirt which stops you sleeping on your back.

Sleep Apnea

If your sleep problems include loud snoring, you stop breathing during your sleep, or you regularly wake up with a sore or dry throat and a morning headache then you may have sleep apnea[60]. If you wake up in the night gasping for breath, or are tired upon waking, find it hard to focus during the day, indeed, find it hard to stay awake then you are most certainly a candidate. See your doctor. This is serious. People with untreated severe sleep apnea usually find a way to die early, mostly from heart attack or stroke. *The plus side is that you won't run out of money in your retirement.*

There are two types of Sleep Apnea: Obstructive[61] and Central.

Obstructive is where the fatty tissues in the mouth and neck slacken as you sleep and constrict your airway. This turns off the air supply to your lungs and sets off your CO_2 alarm, as if you have been holding your breath under water too long. Your body panics and wakes you up enough to breathe again. Blood pressure and heart rate spike, your oxygen levels drop;

it's all nasty. And it may happen thirty times a night, or even thirty times an hour.

Central is where your brain forgets to tell you how to breathe and is mostly the result of heart condition or stroke. We will not deal with the rare Central Sleep Apnea here, since it is doubtful that you would still be working in the aviation game.

Obstructive Sleep Apnea

If you smoke you are *three times* more likely to have it than people who have never smoked. And as soon as you stop smoking the risk begins to plummet. Also, like snoring; alcohol, tranquillizers, sleeping pills can be a factor. If you are a man you are more likely to get it than women. Two for one. Although women's risk increases after menopause.

If you are overweight, and specifically if your body mass index is 30 or greater, your chance of having it starts to rise. Once again you can thank your parents (especially if you are skinny and have it), because you have inherited a fat neck and thin airways.

Congestion is another cause, either by allergy, illness or such things as inflated adenoids, uvula or tonsils, or if you have a deviated-septum (the airways within your nose are crooked or blocked).

Once you reach sixty years you reach the danger zone.

Here's how you reach seventy: **see a Doctor**.

Get into a sleep study[62]. Either at a sleep clinic or, more available nowadays, you can perform a test at home. Here your heart rate, oxygen level, brain activity, breathing rate, flow, and muscle movement are measured, along with the loudness of your snoring. Find out if you have a problem. Treatment can mean a massive increase in the quality of your life perhaps for the first time ever, since sleep apnea even occurs in children.

The fixes are (while you are still young enough):

- Get fit.
- Stop smoking.
- Lose weight.
- Stop drinking alcohol (or cut back to a sensible level).
- Stop taking sleeping pills and tranquillizers.
- Three squirts of Nytol throat spray before sleep which lubricates the throat.
- Using a dental mouth guard which holds your jaw in the right position to sleep.
- Using a jaw bra (you think I am joking?) which does the same thing as the mouth guard but messes up your hair.
- Breathing through a mask that fits over your nose and provides constant air pressure which keeps your airways open. Called a CPAP machine, it is instantly successful. It never cures the problem, only keeps it at bay. For the 50% of people who stop using it within the first year (most within the first month) complaining that it is uncomfortable, they are kidding themselves.
- A recent technology, designed to keep pressure in the airways as you exhale, are the Provent nasal plugs. They have a nifty valve that allows you to breathe in as much as you need. When you

breathe out the valve constricts, providing back-pressure into your airways. It sounds as if it would be difficult to get to sleep, but the manufacturers suggest that you begin sleeping while breathing through your mouth. When you are fully asleep you automatically switch to nose breathing. Who would have thought?

- Another fix is a surgical procedure that places tiny plastic rods in the back of your throat to stiffen the palate, or a laser procedure that burns scars into the same region to have a similar effect. They may be worth a try but not guaranteed a success. After spending the money, and suffering the recovery pain, and STILL having to go to a CPAP machine, patients often report that they would go straight to the CPAP machine if they had their time over.

- An operation called a Tracheotomy *(turn away because this is revolting)*, where they cut a hole in your neck, bypassing the throat, and insert a valve. During the day you can speak and breathe normally; at night, flick the switch and air goes straight into your lungs. Of course it is much more sophisticated than it sounds, and there's little chance that you'd still be flying with this condition.

As with most problems, the expert always tends to use their favorite tools. For carpenters, every problem resembles a nail which is best fixed with a hammer. For preachers, prayer. So what do you think a surgeon is going to suggest?

The *best* fix is this magic pill that you take before sleeping which fixes everything and tastes like chocolate.

It doesn't exist right now but with twelve million Americans diagnosed with sleep apnea and maybe millions more who haven't been diagnosed, you can bet that a huge amount of research is being done at this very moment to find the *Viagra of the throat.*

The bottom line is that if there is a chance you have sleep apnea, get it treated. Don't believe a word of what you have read here. See a professional.

RECAPPING:

Sleep apnea leads to early death. There are two types of sleep apnea *(and only one type of death)***:**

- **Obstructive** (airways)
- **Central** (brain)

Causes (Obstructive):

- **Smoking**
- **Drinking**
- **Taking sleeping pills and tranquillizers**
- **Gender**
- **Obesity**
- **Genetics** (blame your parents)
- **Congestion**
- **Age**

See your doctor and do a sleep test to confirm.

Fixes:

- **Get fit** (playing the Australian Didgeridoo for 25 minutes a day, 6 days a week helped some people).
- **Stop smoking.**
- **Stop drinking.**
- **Stop taking sleeping pills and tranquillizers.**
- **Lose weight.**
- **Use a sleep aid** (throat spray, dental, jaw bra or nose plugs).
- **Use a CPAP machine.**
- **Have an airway strengthening operation.**
- **Have a tracheotomy and** *snorkel when you sleep.*

Further reading:

- Nytol Spray[63]
- CPAP Machines[64]
- Provent Nasal Plugs[65]

Stress

Anything that can be regarded as stressful can have an effect on how well you sleep. Even favorable events in your life can add stress. We know that ulcers and heart problems are exacerbated by stress, but there is significant knowledge to suggest that the body's ability to fight disease, even cancer, is affected by the amount of stress in one's life. After sorting out the clinical aspect of their disease, cancer patients are taught to share their problem in a group, undertake meditation and yoga.

Every survey on stress is highly reported by newspaper editors. Having a relaxing weekend lie-in? Turn to the newspaper's magazine section and read about how stressed you are. The reports point out that 25-40% of stress is caused by your work (or lack of it), and 25-40% is caused by your finances (or lack of them). Throw in the spouse, in-laws, your kids and what the neighbors think and it's wondrous that you have made it this far.

Who knows, or cares, about the masses? It's *your* personal stress that counts, and how you deal with it.

You can thank your forebears for your ability to rise to stressful situations. Mostly it's genetic, and if they weren't good at it, they would have been eaten by a sabre tooth tiger and you wouldn't be here. The mere fact that you are reading this means that you have quality genes.

Stress can help us to achieve great things. We've all heard of sportspeople, actors and television presenters who throw-up before performing. I have even worked with a cabin crew who threw-up after takeoff on every flight (hi Deb). None of them have been fazed by it, and all have performed well once the action starts. In Deb's case, she handled an actual runway excursion, crash and disembarkation without a passenger being injured. She's the crew member you'd want to have beside you in an emergency; even if she had just filled the sick bag.

And don't forget the lottery winners. A cursory glance on the web features thousands of gloating articles about people who went from rags to riches and back to the gutter again. Winners of large amounts of money have a 70% chance of returning to financial obscurity after one hell of a ride, it seems. And aren't we, the losers, happy about that? Newspaper editors seem to think we are.

I witnessed a wise engineer (he invented and marketed the 44 gallon drum rotisserie BBQ) win Victoria's Tattslotto by himself one week. He then shared first prize with about twelve others only three weeks later. Who says no-one ever wins twice? He bought the hotel in his favorite hamlet, bought his wife the general store and the service station for his daughter and mechanic husband. At the pub we'd have to listen to him play the Wurlitzer organ during Sunday lunch.

Despite their enthusiasm and pleasant natures, the family eventually lost the lot. Instead of working themselves to death, they should have invested the lot and drawn a stipend of 4% a year. They would have lived well and never touched the capital. Instead they were super-stressed, trying to do the right thing by everybody and helped no-one in the long run, except the real estate agent and a lawyer or two.

At one of my airlines (there have been a few), pilots were asked to fill-in the *Holmes and Rahe Stress Test*. Ticking "Death of a spouse or family member," admitting to a "divorce," "large home loan," and "Christmas" earned the response: "Do Not Operate Heavy Machinery!" which drew a few smiles around the crew room before we headed off to fly. It doesn't take much to put you in the red band.

If your life has been fairly stress-free then major events will stop you sleeping, but the human brain soon adapts and you will find others who have artery-busting stress levels sleeping like babies. Until the day they never wake up.

Learning to recognize your stress factors is important. Having seen your enemy, it is easier to deal with it. The best way is to discover where you sit on the Holmes and Rahe Stress Scale which can be found on the internet. I use the one on the MindTools website.

Having realized you are potentially in trouble do this:

- Do not make big decisions.
- Write down what the issues are.
- Share your problem, immediately; one of your friends may offer a suggestion or a point of view that is helpful. It is always clearer to see the way out of someone else's problems, rather than your own.

Decide which stress factors can be shed, best done during a session with a pad and pencil, using the models below:

- Plus / Minuses List
- SWOT Analysis
- Urgent / Important Matrix

Amazingly, and especially if you do the exercise with a helpful friend or trained counsellor, the solution jumps off the page at you. In days you could be looking back wondering what the fuss was about. Eventually you will be hard-pressed to remember which year it occurred.

Plus / Minuses List

Rule a line down the middle of a sheet of paper. At the top of the page on the left write PLUS, and at the top of the page on the right write MINUS. Then list the pros and cons of the situation to visualize the benefits of continuing or changing a course of action.

Some people then score each point with a number (out of ten) and arrive at an overall result *(Green eyes may attract **+6**, live-in mother-in-law may score a **-10**.)* For problems of a subjective nature another column may be added "Feelings / Interests" to allow a number to be attributed to how the decision will make you feel.

SWOT analysis

Objectively examine the issue causing stress and address each facet to your personality or situation. It may be a simple way of helping you identify a wise course of action.

Strengths
I am presentable, hard worker, deep thinker.
I could do this new job well.

Weaknesses
Not good at numbers, or public speaking.
Takes people time to realize that I am not just "slow".

Opportunities

Can do an online course on spreadsheets, which can hide my lack of arithmetical skills.

Can join Toastmasters and/or explore YouTube courses on verbal presentation.

Can explore getting a mentor, someone successful in business who knows the real me, to take me under their wing and give advice and contacts.

Threats

One of my competitors for the role appears to have all the goods. But he's sure to be deficient in one or more areas, therefore it's up to me to find out as much as I can about him to see if I can discover his weakness, and neutralize my negative self-talk.

SWOT analyses are helpful from personal matters to large corporate and government decisions. Threats are traditionally things over which you have no control that may affect your business, *'Government may ban suntan lounges,'* necessitating a back-up business plan.

Urgent / Important Matrix

The four square matrix is the most helpful tool when you are feeling super-stressed because of demands on your time, when you are feeling pulled from every direction, lacking sleep, and feeling like you are only surviving with no end in sight.

Draw a large square. Now whack a huge plus sign in the middle, dividing it into four equal squares to make it look like this:

NOT URGENT IMPORTANT	URGENT IMPORTANT
NOT URGENT NOT IMPORTANT	URGENT NOT IMPORTANT

NOT URGENT, IMPORTANT.
"I have to pay my car registration before the end of
the month"

URGENT, IMPORTANT.
"I have to pay my car registration before 5pm
today"

NOT URGENT, NOT IMPORTANT
"I have to pay Mike's car registration before the
end of the month"

URGENT, NOT IMPORTANT
"I have to pay Mike's car registration before
5pm today"

Now, despite what your father told you about
paying bills (he was the son of a Depression Era father
so his thinking is biased) the difference between paying
your car registration now, when you get the bill, or at
the end of the month is negligible. Your bank, or
theirs, who cares? Leaving the money in your account
is not going to make you even ten cents interest. If you
pay it now, or in the next day or two when you are
doing your accounts, rather than in thirty-five days, it

means nothing. It's NOT URGENT, but it is IMPORTANT. If you don't pay it you don't drive.

If you leave it until the day it's due, you can't go the movies or out to lunch; you can't do anything until you pay it. And now it's too late to mail, you have to take to their office personally. It's URGENT and IMPORTANT. It's so stressful that you can't even complete a thought until it is done.

Mike asks you to pay his car registration before the end of the month. We all know someone like him. He breezes through life, charming people to do stuff for him. He has a knack of picking the go-fers who think nothing of appeasing him. *(He would never try it on me, for he knows my response in advance).* Paying his car registration by the end of the month is NOT URGENT and, to you, NOT IMPORTANT. Worse is when he rings you up from his beach house and pleads with you to help him by paying his car registration TODAY so he can drive home tomorrow. It's URGENT but, to you, NOT IMPORTANT.

The trick in life is to rule a big black line right across the page, halfway down; and for everything that is NOT IMPORTANT you:

"Smile and say NO"

You **must**, however, **offer a solution**.

Like this:

'I'd love to Mike, but I am busy right now. I can't do it for you … but how about Julie? I know she is looking for pocket money, I am sure she'd love to run into the city for you. Here is her number…'

Then shut up.

The key to sales negotiation is

"He who speaks first loses."

Having made your closing statement and request for the order, you say nothing, instead imagine eating a juicy apple. Mike can't help but fill the dead-air with words, eventually muttering :

'*OK, thank you.*'

After a couple of times he will stop asking you.

Until you get your life back under control, ONLY concentrate on things that are important to you personally. Concentrate on moving everything that is URGENT into the NOT URGENT box. Soon you will get a reputation for being the person who has all the answers, without doing anything for anyone, except directing traffic and smiling all the time.

The system even works for family situations.

Your aging mother is not good at paying her bills. It stresses her. Which stresses you. When you are visiting, steal all the utility and phone bills and, in your time, put them onto direct debit with your bank account. Unless she has a boyfriend she rings in Paris, it will be a small amount of money well spent. If you normally do her shopping, go online and set up her weekly shop and monthly restock with her local supermarket. Time the deliveries for the two hour window when you'll be there. You'll still be doing all the things for your mother but when it fits into your schedule, and at last you will feel in control.

Using these tools to recognize the problem won't help you sleep better; you need a plan of attack before your brain will turn off. Brainstorm for solutions with some mind-mapping.

Mind-Maps

There are some excellent software packages available which are helpful for collaborative teams (and priced accordingly) but nothing is more satisfying than sitting up in bed in the morning sunshine with a cup of tea, a large artists pad (10 pages 290 gsm art paper) and a few fine-tipped markers. In the center of the page write the problem, for example: EXPENSIVE CAR LOAN and draw a fluffy cloud around it. All around the cloud write words as they come to you and connect them by lines to the central cloud and to each other if they link.

This brainstorming is meant to be creative; throw the words down as they come to you, it's not meant to be pretty (you can make a pretty one later). Significant thoughts might get their own cloud.

In this case some surrounding clouds may be:

- Sell The Car
- Refinance The Car with a Cheaper Loan
- Get A Second Job

Position other thoughts as they come to you and connect with lines. Here you may use different colors to follow different threads.

Sprouting around 'Sell the Car' you might add:

- Find out the loan payout figure
- Check out the market price
- Get the car serviced
- Get the car cleaned up for sale
- Decide: dealer or private sale

Sprouting from 'private sale' you might add:

- Take photos
- Internet ad
- Choose date
- Ask Uncle John if we can do the test drives/ presentations at his place

SMART Decisions

From these brain-play options will come some decisions. These become apparent and are hit with the highlighter.

We will make sure they don't die on the paper by ensuring that each one is S.M.A.R.T. and condensed into bite size actions (deliverables) which have to be done by a certain person, by certain a date.

S.M.A.R.T. means:
- Specific
- Measurable
- Achievable
- Realistic
- Time Bound

Before we decide if we have to sell the car in the above example, we must decide if "Refinancing the Car with a Cheaper Loan" is not easier and faster to achieve. For example:

Specific

Ring the finance company, speak to a loans officer and ask how we can get the payments down $150 a month by refinancing with a lower interest rate, extending the loan term and/or increasing the balloon payout figure.

Measurable

We'll know when we have a dollar amount answer.

Achievable

Yes, I have the guy's business card from when I bought the car. I can ring at lunch time tomorrow.

Realistic

Sure. I have a good credit record, and a steady job. This tough patch is lasting longer than I'd like. I am a good customer. Looking after me is easier for him than trying to find a new customer.

Time Bound

I give myself until Wednesday evening to get an answer. Thursday we decide on selling the car.

Dealing with stressors, making decisions, gives you a great sense of control and empowerment. Emptying your brain before you go to bed allows you to sleep easily.

As well, your subconscious is a perfect problem-solver while you sleep. Once you have defined the three choices:

- Sell The Car?
- Refinance The Car with a Cheaper Loan?
- Get A Second Job?

and have written them out before you go to bed, the chances are that when you wake, after the first restful sleep in ages, the correct answer is clear in your mind:

"Sell the car, and buy a cheap runabout for cash. Then hire an expensive car when I want to do a long weekend road trip because realistically, it's only once every six months."

The internet is full of websites devoted to this topic, one which does the trick is Mindtools.com[66]

RECAPPING:

- Do the Holmes and Rahe Stress Scale.
- If you are stressed:
    - Do not make big decisions
    - Write down what the issues are
    - Share your problem with someone you trust
- Determine the important stress factors
    - Plus / Minuses List
    - SWOT Analysis, and
    - Urgent / Important Matrix
- Get creative using
    - Mind-Maps to discover options, then
    - Make S.M.A.R.T. decisions

- Write the list of possible decisions before you sleep and let your subconscious choose.

From the Logbook

Shelley was the human face of the increasing productivity of the aviation industry. She was one of three personal secretaries sitting outside the CEO's office. The new CEO arrived who was not only capable of using his own computer, but he could type at 40 words per minute. In a flash, secretaries became as extinct as dinosaurs, even twenty-three year old ones.

She had been placed in the "HR pool" where she was used by various project teams before being made redundant. While she was assisting me during an eight month project, I became aware of the *"Sword of Damocles"* hanging over her desk by a thread. One day after lunch, I saw her race back to her desk, tears welling, grab her handbag and race out the door.

By the time I finished my phone call and rang her mobile it was about twelve to fifteen minutes. Through sobs she declared that she had heard the consultants talking in the corridor, that they would be "letting her go" at the end of the week.

'I was so upset, I just took off!'

Thinking she had gone down to the canteen I was confused because I couldn't hear the usual canteen background noise and asked where she was. She was home! In a matter of minutes she had left the office block, gone to the car park across the busy six lane street, retrieved her car, and driven home. The fastest she could normally drive home was fifteen minutes, not including time to get to, or even out of, the carpark. When I asked her which way she had driven home, she couldn't tell me. She had no idea.

Another major stressor was that her favorite grandfather had recently died.

No-one knows how each of us will react to an extreme stress event. In Shelley's case the FLIGHT response took over. Luckily she didn't kill herself or anyone else.

After my father died I didn't think I was in shock.

I don't remember signing the documents for the legal class action to recover money lost due to a failed investment. Yet, there was my signature, so I must have. I seem to remember someone saying that there were 128 investors in the action.

Turns out there were about five who were in the class action. And we had to pay all the legal fees of an expensive law firm, unless we could convince the other 123 investors to also join the class action. So began six of the worst years of my life.

When you have a life stress event do not sign any documents.

After 9/11, twenty-eight airlines around the world went broke, their aircraft loans far outweighing the value of their planes. Ours was among them. A Boeing 727, if you could find a buyer, was worth about $10,000. But there were no buyers. The Mojave Desert graveyard for used airplanes was full of them.

My mind-mapping exercise ran to three pages, two columns each, of an A4 legal pad, listing all the things that I *could* turn my hand to. About sixty things.

I have since done three of them.

When you have received such a kick in the guts, the mind-map process gives you confidence to get up and have another go at life. Invaluable.

I still have those yellowed pages. And who knows? Maybe one day I will be "A Radio Operator In The Antarctic Expedition" after all … *the Morse Code at 15 words per minute that I learned to obtain my Air Transport Pilot's License has to be good for something.*

Do not make ANY major decisions during times of stress. Trust the experts, if their Stress Scale says you are most likely stressed, believe them.

Talk to your doctor about it and take time to recover. It may be brand new to you, but doctors see this all the time and are trained to get you to the other end safely.

Sun - Too Much

My sister, a doctor on her way to becoming a dermatologist, announced to our family dinner table that only four major sunburns in your life was enough to give you skin cancer. Our party-girl mother paused serving the vegetables long enough to wave the serving-spoon at the three of us kids, and declared:

'Then you lot are dead!'

She was referring to the fact that our childhood summers were spent in the harsh Australian sun.

The extent of our protection was a dab of white zinc cream on the nose. Few Australians of my age have their noses chopped-off, but my sister and her colleagues have made careers of removing bits of their countrymen on a regular basis. They'll have a go at tourists too. The visible equatorial Sun, wandering between the tropics of Cancer and Capricorn as the planet navigates its way around our favorite star on an inclination of 23.5 degrees, is a known killer; but my Mum's remarks were pointing to the dangerous *southern* Sun.

We were discovering that every squirt of underarm deodorant, hairspray, insect spray, air freshener, and fire extinguisher was releasing CFCs (a word too big to remember) that whizzed up to the stratosphere and damaged the ozone layer. So much so that a "hole" opened up in the Antarctic spring of the early 1980s, and ozone levels dropped by 60%. The precious layer sits about twenty-three kilometers up (80,000 feet), twice the height that jetliners fly, and it's here the rare ozone molecule protects earth from ultra violet radiation.

How rare? Very rare. Take ten million air molecules. Within that are two million oxygen molecules. And only THREE ozone molecules. Or about 0.6 parts per million of our atmosphere.

The hole opens and closes with the seasons. The Montreal Protocol, effective as of 1987, banned the use of CFCs and while the damage peaked in 1997, the hole should be repaired within fifty years according to the Daily Mail's report on the UN Environment Programme & World Meteorological Organization[67].

The Ozone Layer is charged by lightning, most notably in the Catatumbo Lightning storms in Venezuela (which contributes 25% of the planet's upper level ozone production) and by storms above a village called Kifuka in the Democratic Republic of the Congo (which must be an exciting place to live).

Worldwide, the planet experiences forty-four lightning strikes per second (+/- 5). That's over 3.8 million a day. Without them we would be dead. Only 25% of lightning strikes hit the ground as most are contained within or between clouds. And lightning produces ozone. Your nose is even sensitive enough to smell it.

Under this widening ozone hole, we were lying on the beach, reading James Bond novels, smoking, and working on our tans. For boys this meant doing nothing except trying to look cool. The girls, however, were basting themselves with Baby Oil (I still can't get my head around that name) or coconut oil. You could almost hear the sizzling.

It was particularly unfair to the Tasmanians, Kiwis, and those south of Santiago and Buenos Aires in South America. Not only did they freeze in winter, suffering the short, cold days of those who live close to the poles, but the sun, when they saw it, was frying them alive. Areas lacking the protection of the healthy ozone layer also notice an increase in cases of cataracts to the eyes. It is a common operation in the elderly. Plus, in areas devoid of ozone above, plant crops fail.

We seriously need the stuff.

The danger of too much sun is known, and there is a great deal of research about it if you need convincing. We have lost hundreds of sportspeople, actors, and performers to skin cancers. Bob Marley and Eva Cassidy to name two, plus a brave young Australian called Clare Oliver whose campaign against tanning lounges may change the world.

"A healthy tan" ... isn't.

Culturally, Asian cultures favor lighter skin. Beaches in Vietnam are littered with Europeans sun-baking, while the locals sit under hundreds of overlapping beach umbrellas. The Russians trying to get brown and the Vietnamese trying to get white. On your next visit to Asia, try buying skin moisturizer without "lightener" or "whitener" added. Good luck.

When it comes to the nasties, it's the ultraviolet that gets you. It is predictable based on your location on the planet, the time of day, and day of the year, even if there are high level clouds. On sun-tanning beds it doesn't matter what time of year it is. One unnoticed skin cancer cell, and you are dead. This is why Australians now get their skin checked once or twice a year.

When my sister messaged me from a conference in Iceland declaring that there had been a skin cancer spike in that country's airline pilots, she wondered about cockpits. I wrote back:

'Have you ever seen an Air Icelandic crew beside the pool in Bahrain?'

The days of three day layovers, heavy partying, no sun-screen and crippling sunburn are over for most airline crews. But not our passengers. Flying English tourists to and from the Greek Islands one summer I greeted one of our returning passengers who looked as if she had spent three days tending a blast furnace wearing a bikini.

'This is nothing! You wait 'til you see Sharon. She was in the hospital for three days! Fantastic holiday ... we're coming back next year!'

Which sums-up too much sun.

Use an app if you are travelling. Know your latitude (and hemisphere), check the U.V. weather reports and use a SPF15 moisturizer every day between summer equinoxes:

- From March 21st until September 21st in the northern hemisphere, and

- From September 21st until March 21st in the southern hemisphere.

Don't go out for more than twenty minutes in the direct sun without covering up anytime your shadow is shorter than yourself. That is, from about 9 a.m. 'til 4 p.m. between the summer equinoxes. And follow the guidelines recommended by the experts[68] [69]

Why?

Because despite losing your sight, having my sister chop and freeze bits off you, along with the chance that you could be dead in six weeks from skin cancer, it is not easy to *sleep* when you have had too much sun.

After a soothing shower, slicing a chilled Aloe Vera plant open and smearing the gel over sunburned skin aids sleep better than the commercial preparations. If no plant is available make sure that the Aloe Vera content of moisturizer is more than just 'flavoring.'

RECAPPING:

- Too much sun exposure is bad for you as it can cause skin cancer.

- Get your skin checked. Every year.

- Any changes to a mole or mark on your skin must be investigated.

- Death can come quickly from skin cancer.

- Your location on the planet, and proximity to the Ozone Holes, have a bearing on the amount of safe exposure.

- Use moisturizer with SP15 every day between the equinoxes over summer.

- Sunburn is to be avoided as it prevents restful SLEEP.

From the Logbook

During my first visit to the Australian State of Queensland there was a huge billboard exclaiming

"One in three Queenslanders will get skin cancer."

I wiped my brow and muttered:

'Thank God I come from Victoria.'

There was also a sign in Brisbane which has nothing at all to do with sleeping but tickles me to this day:

"Metropolitan Funerals - Customer Parking Only"

Sun - Too Little

Not enough sun. Seasonal Affective Disorder (S.A.D.)

The opposite of the sun-tanned, crispy, crackling old person (no wait, they only look old) is the white pasty man who has not left the confines of his basement for the last ten years. One friend calls this type "the computer stinky." Unwashed, unhealthy, living by the light of the screen, only emerging to restock beer, Coca-Cola and cigarettes.

If you want to see this breed congregate take a trip to Bangkok Airport and hang out at the baggage carrousel of any European flight during the northern winter. Men with *Introverted Personality Disorder* are on their way to meet the lady of their dreams, or so they think. Spending your waking hours online does not make you attractive to the opposite sex, no matter how comparatively rich you are. They are not all Norwegians (mostly from the U.K. and Germany), but they are trying to use the Norwegian system for beating the S.A.Ds (Seasonal Affective Disorders) caused by lack of sunlight.

According to the witty Lorelou Desjardins, a French lady who has relocated to Norway, the Norwegians' secret weapon is the **S.A.S. 'Sex, Alcohol & Syden** (which translates as "the south"). Her hilarious website,

A Frog in the Fjord, is mandatory reading on the subject. In her article, **"How to survive your winter depression[70]"** she says that, ideally, you should snuggle up with someone, use alcohol to make them appealing or, better still, head south for winter. If this sounds extreme, try a Norwegian winter, or any winter where you are at your desk before the sun comes up and still there when the sun goes down. You'll soon understand.

Seasonal Affective Disorder is a real depressive illness. It's genetic to an extent, so if you noticed your mom and dad getting drunk and retiring to the bedroom before slipping out to the Bahamas each winter, chances are it may affect you too. As you hibernate your way through winter, S.A.D. ensures you will put on weight and even sleep longer than normal, though not well. We all do it to some degree when the weather's cold and bleak by seeking out starchy comfort food such as hearty soups, lamb shanks with mashed potato, followed by hot sticky date pudding. It's even worth traveling to Warsaw in winter to experience Zapiecek Restaurant's Russian Dumplings followed by Potato Pancakes covered in Hungarian Goulash accompanied by their hot mulled-wine. In winter we eat too many calories. It's cold and dark, and wet, we get less exercise (you can see this coming can't you?) then we get fat.

The symptoms of S.A.D:

Feeling lethargic, lacking in energy, not interested in physical contact (you're overweight and the concept of someone running their hands over your flab is unappealing), anxious, irritable, and unable to cope.

Even depression.

The medical websites suggest that you see your doctor to make sure it isn't anything more serious. For me, instead of giving my doctor money for a small chat,

I might try fixing myself by spending it on alcohol, sex, and a flight to the tropics.

I know how to fix my depression, by "taking the black dog for a walk in the morning." No-one on the planet, no matter how bad they have felt, has felt worse after a morning walk (unless they were hit by a car). Especially if accompanied by a puppy.

Force yourself to get up and do your daily exercise in the sunshine.

No sun?

Consider using light therapy.

Get a bright white light, with as little ultra violet as possible, put it close to your face (about twenty centimeters, or eight inches) for an hour every morning before 8 a.m. The newer LED light boxes need only be used for about thirty minutes to achieve the same effect. The trick, it seems, is to have the light in front and slightly above you. And to do the treatment every day. In one study it wasn't until close to four weeks before the light treatment patients started feeling noticeably better than the control group. Some suggest that it doesn't hurt to have a negative ion generator working nearby at the same time.

The Mayo Clinic suggests that light treatment is effective and has more detailed information than is needed here. Light boxes are available online. You want no blue light, and preferably L.E.D. If I lived in a such a northern location (and the alcohol/sex/tropical option was not available), I would get a walking treadmill, rig-up the light and ion generator, plug in audiobooks and walk half an hour a day.

While some people suffering S.A.D sleep less during the winter months, with the increased darkness there is a tendency to sleep longer. If you find oversleeping makes you wake feeling irritable, try setting your alarm to wake after eight hours and note the difference.

Vitamin D

Having a deficiency of Vitamin D is another by-product of a vampire lifestyle, which could be a cause muscle weakness, and pain deep in your bones.

It is said that Vitamin D deficiency can be associated with

- Rickets
- Cardiovascular disease
- Cognitive impairment
- Cancer
- Severe asthma in children

To make things scarier, an internet search also mentions diabetes, hypertension, glucose intolerance *and* multiple sclerosis.

(What about Poverty and The Plague too? Sometimes it's better if you don't look at the medical websites.)

This we know: you are more likely to be deficient in Vitamin D if you are:

1) A vegan.

Eggs, fish, cod liver oil and fortified milk are a source of Vitamin D. If you are not consuming these you may have a problem.

2) Someone who gets little (or no) sun.

Only ten minutes sunshine a day, on your skin, can give you enough Vitamin D. You should get no more than fifteen minutes of exposure in areas with high UV exposure.

3) Someone who has dark skin, which has less ability to make the vitamin from sun exposure.

This is where you *do* want to go and visit your doctor. Next time you are there ask for a blood test for Vitamin D. You will most likely find that your current lifestyle is getting you enough. And yes, you can take an expensive pill, but is it as effective as the Vitamin D collected from nature? My theory on vitamin pills is that each one is an admission that your lifestyle is deficient and it's best to treat your body to the real stuff.

Finally, before going to press these latest research results were announced, tipping the whole topic on its head.

An extensive study conducted by Dr. Erin S. LeBlanc[71] and others concluded:

"We found <u>no evidence</u> that treating Vitamin D deficiency decreased risk for:
- *Fracture*
- *Cancer*
- *Diabetes*
- *Or that it improved:*
- *Psychosocial, or*
- *Physical health"*

Either way, hedging your bets, a bit of sunshine every day isn't going to hurt.

RECAPPING:

- **Consider if you are suffering the S.A.Ds, and decide if it's something you should see your doctor about.** (See the Stress chapter).
- **Use the Norwegian method: sex, alcohol and visit the South** (That'd be the North if you're *Down-Under*)
- **Daily exercise.**
- **And/or light therapy.**
- **See your doctor and get a blood test for Vitamin D to see if you are deficient.**
- **If your results are low, increase your fish and egg intake, or cod liver oil.**
- **Get ten minutes of sunshine on your skin a day.**
- **Try to live without Vitamin D pills by modifying your lifestyle.**

Water

Imagine a wonder drink which could help you[72]:

- increase energy,
- relieve fatigue,
- lose weight,
- flush out toxins,
- improve your skin complexion, and
- "regularity",
- boost your immune system,
- prevent headaches,
- cramps and sprains, and
- put you in a good mood.

Most of all, it can help you sleep better. Available anywhere. Water.

It should be worth bottling.

In fact, Craig Zucker did just that, and charged Californians $1.50 per bottle of New York tap water under the name "Tap'D NY."

Those who are into the stuff prefer to pay more than double the price of gas, or 2,000 times the price of tap water to get the bottle with the blue cap. A liter of which required 1.39 liters of water to make[73]. One day wars will be fought over the stuff. It is more important than oil. For without it, you're disabled after three days and dead before eight.

In March 2014 the United Nations[74] reported that:

"At the end of 2011, an estimated 768 million people did not use an improved source for drinking-water.

Ten countries are home to two-thirds of the global population without access to improved drinking water sources:

China   (108 million)
India   (99 million)
Nigeria   (63 million)
Ethiopia   (43 million)
Indonesia   (39 million)
Democratic Republic of the Congo   (37 million)
Bangladesh   (26 million)
United Republic of Tanzania   (22 million)
Pakistan   (16 million)
Kenya   (16 million)

Diarrheal diseases linked to a lack of safe water, sanitation, and basic hygiene, kills approximately 1,400 children under five every day. This amounts to over half a million children per year.

In Africa alone, people spend forty billion hours every year just walking to collect water. Women carry two thirds of the burden in drinking water collection, leaving less time for other socioeconomic activities.

Girl's school attendance increased significantly for every hour reduction in water collection. For example, in Nepal attendance recently improved by over 30%."

While people are literally dying to get hold of clean drinking water in Asia and Africa, western societies are full of people who turn-up their noses at the stuff.

But that'd be a mistake.

Adding sugar and caffeine, in fact, adding anything to water is pretty stupid and does little good. In fact, it mostly does harm. Your body needs about 3 liters a day for men and 2.2 liters a day for women. 20% comes from your food, if you are eating your vegetables.

Drinks provide most of your hydration, although coffee, tea, soft drinks, and alcohol mostly act as *diuretics*, that is to say that they increase the amount of urine, defeating the purpose. Despite the number cups of coffee and green tea you drink a day, you still need to drink plain water to get adequate hydration. If you were sitting doing nothing you'd need about 100ml (3.3 ounces) per hour. Good hydration means that you rarely feel thirsty, urinate about 1.5 liters a day and the urine is almost clear. If you feel thirsty, you are becoming dehydrated. Drink now. If you are excessively thirsty it may be a sign of diabetes, see your doctor.

Want to see the difference water makes?

Search the internet for images for before and after eight weeks of hydration and note the reduction of lines around eyes and general healthiness of the skin. Some people claim a reduction in cellulite marks, some have lost weight. You will note that people often add make-up to their after shots, defeating the purpose; go one better and make your own set of photos.

Sports Drinks

The biggest marketing con is to get anyone undertaking a normal fitness routine to pay for special "sports drinks." They quote faster rates of absorption as selling points, but the normal absorption rate of water is spectacular anyway, and can be discounted for average humans. While the salts and electrolytes contained in sports drinks are definitely required for serious athletes (you know who you are) they are a waste of time if you are doing less than sixty minutes of normal exercise at a time.

Rule of thumb, before you go out on your walk, drink a glass of water. Then drink one when you come back. If you are hot and sweaty, have another. 300ml (10oz) per half hour is what you need, which amounts to an average glass in the kitchen cupboard. Yes, there are people who have died from drinking too much water (it's called drowning); sorry, Hyponatremia (too little salt) which may be an issue for endurance athletes, ecstasy-fueled clubbers, and people trying to win a bet. Stay below four liters evenly-spaced in twenty-four hours and you should be alive to tell the tale.

Airborne

Funnily, cabin crew complain that being in aircraft at altitude dries out their skin and then proceed to not drink enough water. Most airlines gives each pilot a 1.2 liter bottle of water each duty period which we see as a challenge to finish. Sipping almost constantly to finish the bottle in the last half hour before the last landing results in less fatigue for the approach, a clear head and sand-free eyes for touchdown. Though after taxi-in, during disembarkation, there is often a race for the loo, (in my airline the cabin crew stick huge bags of blankets in there for a joke).

Hotels

For hotel dwellers, the industry is vague as to the quality of its water. One would imagine that the treatment plants within five star hotels means that you can drink straight out of the cold tap. But there is no readily accessible standard. If your hotel room has free bottles of water in the bathroom, then you shouldn't trust the tap water. If it has glasses in the bathroom, assume it's OK. If in doubt, call reception and ask.

A good sign is to smell the chlorine. That means that the hotel (if not the city) has decided to kill the nasties by use of chlorine, an excellent method. Chlorine is safe to drink up until four parts per million, and one part per million is enough to kill the Giardia Protozoan (the common cause of diarrhea) in forty-five minutes. As a side note, if you ever have to disinfect water, add two drops of unscented household bleach per liter of water and wait an hour. If you are really doing this, why not add four drops? Bleach breaks down over time and chances are the bottle under the sink is not fresh.

When entering hotel rooms, if you are worried about the chlorinated water, a trick is to fill every glass in the place with cold water. As chlorine is about 1.5 times heavier than water, even though it is boiled into a gas at -40C (-40F), it remains in your water. Go down to meet the crew at the bar and by the time you get back you can happily drink the top 7/8ths of every glass knowing that you are getting nothing but clean pure water. The chemicals are at the bottom of the glass. In places with dodgy air-conditioning crew will tell you that they fill the bath and hand basin to get some moisture into the atmosphere. They complain of dry skin and sinuses and headaches. They could save the effort by drinking enough water during the day and having a shower before bed.

Sleeping

Now you are an adult, want to save money, look great and you want to live a long time. Drink water. Get over the taste and drink water. It's as important as blood and air. Save the space in your fridge for high quality champagnes, wines and mixers rather than sugary soft drinks or processed juices. And drink water.

Until an hour before bed.

Since you have become fully hydrated, a sip before you sleep is all you need. And you shouldn't find yourself having to get up in the middle of the night. *Well, not after the first week.*

RECAPPING:

- **Water is good for you.**
- **Drink three liters a day (men) and at least two liters a day (women).**
- **Sports drinks are a waste of money for most people.**
- **Anything added to water, (tea, coffee, sugar, cordial etc.) reduces its effectiveness.**
- **Chlorine (bleach) kills evil things in water then settles to the bottom.**
- **Urine should be straw colored in the morning, and clear by the evening.**
- **If you are thirsty you are already dehydrated.**
- **Well-hydrated humans sleep better.**

Further Reading:

The Water Initiative[75]. Delivering water filter systems at point of delivery for 30% of the cost of competitors.

The book *"Abundance: The Future Is Better than You Think"* by Peter H. Diamandis and Steven Kotler (2012) has an inspirational chapter "Water" which shows how easy it is to provide clean drinking water to a planet of 9 billion people. (Audiobook[76] or Amazon[77] Printed Book)

While you're at it, you must read their follow-up book: *"Bold: How to Go Big, Create Wealth and Impact the World."*

Weight (and Sex)

There is a direct correlation between weight and sleep quality. You most likely know this, but if you're not sleeping right the chances are that your weight is not right either. There could be simple reasons why you put on weight if you have not been getting enough sleep. The fact that you are awake longer means you are likely to eat more food, ingesting more calories. Sleeping less than six hours per night causes you to increase weight[78].

Newspaper USA Today[79] reported on a Columbia University study which revealed:

'... *those who get less than four hours sleep have obesity rates 73% higher than those who sleep seven to nine hours; and those who sleep five to six hours are 50% more likely to be obese.*[80]'

In one study, women who slept for six hours or less (or longer than nine hours) put on 5 kg (11 lbs) more compared to women who slept for seven hours per night over one year. That's a significant number.

Not only does it affect how you put ON weight, but also how you LOSE it. In 2011 Dr. Charles Elder from Kaiser Permanent Health Research Center[81] revealed that you double your weight loss if you sleep between six and eight hours sleep each night. If you want to lose weight a great idea is to get proper sleep. But it's hard to sleep well if you are overweight.

Let's tackle the weight first.

Being overweight specifically increases your chances of heart disease, diabetes, and sleeping disorders such as snoring and sleep apnea. Is this news to you? Putting on weight makes you unattractive to your mate, ruins your sex life, makes you unhappy, unfit, unhealthy, causes you to have back pain but most importantly it makes your uniform look like you are the Michelin Man. Passengers are terrified your straining button is going to ping off and hit them in the eye every time you walk past. How do I know?

Because I have broken the springs in scales all around the world, especially when I was working for a Saudi Sheikh flying a VIP A320. One day we went to what we thought was a substantial lunch of every imaginable salad, only to find out later that it was precursor to the main course and desserts.

And I was raised to eat everything on the plate
  ' ... **because of the starving Biafrans.'**
[Digressing, the Republic of Biafra seceded from Nigeria in 1967 until 1970, long enough for one million of its people to be killed in fighting or by starvation. If you are a lapsed Biafran, you will take heart in the knowledge that I ate all my brussel sprouts for you.]

I can say all this because I don't know you. Your family and friends won't tell you. No work colleagues will mention it. Let's face it: you could afford to lose some weight.

Some airlines have a program to ensure that their flight and cabin crew do not become obese. Nifty accountants must have worked out how much it costs to carry a kilo of fat around the skies for one year and have decreed that we should all be much smaller. When you have 10,000 staff all weighing 10 kgs (22 lbs) extra for the men and 5kgs (11 lbs) for the women, it adds up to a significant amount of fuel each year to fly their flab. Uniform re-fittings, days off for health reasons, early retirement due to ill health means that they get less training bang for their buck.

A pilot who urinates in the jar at their medical and fails the diabetes test, costs the business real money. Not to mention, by the way, it also ruins their life. The last landing before today's medical was their last ever, which is a sad way to end your career.

And to be politically incorrect, the airline's passengers also prefer skinny cabin crew to fat ones. How do I know? As soon as people find out you are a pilot you get to hear their entire flying history; and they have told me. Despite my protesting that, during an emergency, you'd be wanting highly-experienced *tubby* crew (like me) I am continually beaten over the head about how crew look and the quality of the on-board service. I have given up arguing.

In 1996 I was holidaying in Singapore and was intrigued to read on the front page of the Straits Times an exposé declaring that prospective cabin crew for Singapore Airlines, during the second round of interviews, *had to parade in front of the board members in swimsuits.*

Knowing that this would provoke a backlash from the readers I eagerly awaited the next day's paper to see how its editor would string the story out, to make it last all week if possible. It was journalistic gold and the advertising manager would be rubbing his hands as he rang *Weight Watchers* and asked if they'd like to buy a full page ad.

Day Two was the predictable tirade from people saying the policy was sexist. The editor never left his office, he probably just asked his male reporters to ring their sisters and write down the abuse.

On Day Three he led with an interview with the airline's CEO, Dr. Cheong Choong Kong, who stated that since 1972 "Singapore Girl" was the face of Singapore, concluding:

'You wouldn't want her to be ugly would you?'

At six a.m. on Day Four I flung open the hotel room door to find my copy of the paper for the next installment. But there was no day four. All readers had, I assume, thoughtfully nodded over their breakfast and answered the airline's CEO:

'No, I wouldn't.'

Nothing more was said. Astounding.

[By 1999 it had changed. A "Singapore Girl" told me that at the second interview they were given black one piece swimsuits to put on, and every inch of their exposed skin was scrutinized by two women. Then they were told to dive in the swimming pool and prove that they could swim. They never had to parade in front of Board Members.]

However, internet rumors abound, from numerous airlines: if you put on significant weight you will be grounded until you *"regain your figure."* So, yes, it's all about image, advertising and marketing; and profits. In an industry where profits are hard to come by.

The UK's Telegraph newspaper reported in September 2015 that Air India had grounded 130 of the 600 cabin crew previously-warned to lose weight[82] and that, in 2013, the airline calculated that by recruiting female cabin crew instead of heavier males they could save GBP 329,000 in fuel costs each year.

A numbers game.

Like weight loss.

Keeping your weight under control is a simple matter of arithmetic. If you put more than 2,000 calories down your throat every day, and only do minimal exercise, you will put on weight.

Excuses like:

- 'I am big boned!'
- 'All our family are large'
- 'I exercise all the time'

might make you feel good. But you are still overweight.

[The 2% of overweight people with real medical issues can stop reading right now, I apologize. See your doctor and good luck with your treatments.]

For the rest of us, tell any story you want. If you have put on weight since you left school then it's due to lifestyle. 2,000 calories a day will keep you at your current weight. You need to reduce your intake if you are going to start eating into your stored reserves.

Cut back on:

- Total food intake
- The dreaded junk food
- Processed food
- Alcohol
- Soft drinks, including anything with "diet" in the name
- Juices
- Sugary fruits
- Sugar
- Chocolate
- Sweets

'What's left?!' I hear you ask, as you begin making a rope noose and search for a tree branch.

There is a fantastic Australian doctor called Dr. John Tickell who can tell you. For years he has been banging-on about fitness, diet and longevity. His first book to grab my attention was the life-changing:

"Laughter, Sex, Vegetables and Fish."

His more recent tome, *'The Great Australian Diet 2'* is worth a look; in this book he has collaborated with his wife (a top fitness instructor) to lead you by the hand and change your life, one day at a time. It includes stories of successful patients who have lost many kilos, each describing their amazing turn around, with astounding before and after photos. It includes tips, exercises and recipes to help you get on track and keep you there as your lifestyle changes.

If you can't wait to read his wisdom on paper, a quick Kindle search, (so you can have him in your life in seconds), reveals his most recent book: *"Love, Laugh, and Eat: And Other Secrets of Longevity from the Healthiest People on Earth."*

Another worthwhile read is "The China Study" which looks at the largest long-term clinical assessment in history, by Campbell, Schurman and Campbell. It marries well with Dan Buettner's *"The Blue Zones"* which is an investigation of places on the planet where people live an abnormally long time. It investigates their locations, their lifestyles and their diets.

In keeping with my late father's theory: 'All knowledge is found in books' I suggest you turn to these books to give you a bedrock foundation of knowledge, not old wives' tales, so you know in your heart what is right and what works. Continue to read inspiring words (or listen to audiobooks) to help steel your resolve as you get your weight down. Simply, the bottom line with all of these studies is:

- Balance calorific intake VS energy expended,
- Embark on doable, daily, physical activity,
- Employ good sleep patterns, and
- Get most of your protein from plants or fish.
- Ditch processed food and junk.

which brings me back to the title of Dr. John's book. You can have as much as you want of Laughter, Sex, Vegetables and Fish ... *but everything else must be in moderation.*

Before embarking on a weight loss campaign see your doctor and get a referral to see a dietitian. As soon as you have two other people working on the problem you will subconsciously not want to let them down. The more people who are helping you in spirit, the easier it becomes.

Discuss a plan of action, set short and long term goals, and agree on key performance indicators. Commit to ninety days in a row to set your new metabolism in stone.

Take BEFORE photos of your body in the mirror. You will soon become staggered at the changes that occur.

Measure your body circumferences with a tape measure. Neck, chest, waist, hips, upper arm, thighs. You are not going to believe these figures in six months, so measure twice.

Work in thirty minutes of exercise a day. New studies reveal that it doesn't even have to be thirty minutes straight, ten minutes before and after work, coupled with a brisk ten minute walk at lunchtime may do the trick.

Saying that you play sports once or twice a week is not exercise. That's sport. Chances are that you spend most of the time watching the action interspersed with short bursts of hamstring-busting action. Then retire to the bar to talk about it and ingest more calories in drinks and bar snacks. Exercise is the "move it or lose it" stuff that you have to do every day. Walking so fast you can hardly speak.

When you wake up in the morning have a large glass of water (see the water chapter). Measure your blood pressure. Measure your weight, and enter these details on a spreadsheet (or exercise book), dates down the left, columns across the top. Subconsciously, you are making a commitment to yourself each day to see a result. Don't worry about daily fluctuations, look at the plateaus and falls over time. Your body is an amazing machine.

Add columns on the spreadsheet to list the amount of exercise that you undertake and also how many glasses of alcohol you take a day. I also list my layover trips as an excuse for gaps in the sheet. List the hours and quality of your sleep. Don't cheat. This is for you, nobody else.

It is surprising how fast you will develop a healthy lifestyle to make the spreadsheet look good. Soon you will be showing it off to your doctor. That's when you know you've turned the corner.

If you are like me, and hate exercise (but do it every day), do the exercise first. Before food, before Facebook, before emails. Plug your audiobook into your ears and get the thirty minutes done. Have a large glass of water before and after the exercise.

Adopt this old premise:
- Breakfast like a King,
- Lunch like Prince, and
- Dine like a Pauper.

Break your fast with a substantial breakfast to reset your metabolism and get things moving. You should eat some fiber. This fast-breaking meal need not be daily at 7 a.m. but what suits your body. If the ideal time for you is ten, that's OK.

Try this:

Microwave some oats in water. Be careful, they explode on a high setting. Try five minutes on 30% power, stir and 30% again. When you have perfected it for your particular mixing bowl and microwave, you can set it as you go out the door to do the exercise. Mine takes nine minutes at 30% power while I am doing my stretches. Mash up some sunflower seeds, walnuts & Brazil nuts. Chuck in a few raisins. (I said *a few*.)

Stir it all up and add a dash a soy milk for consistency. Drizzle a tiny bit of honey over the top to make yourself think you are being naughty.

Slice half a banana (they are full of sugar) OR one small apple and mix it all together.

Do not eat standing up, reading or watching television. Make a big production of eating at a table, savoring each mouthful, chewing everything completely. Use a small spoon and make the meal last a long time. Finish with a cup of hot green tea.

Agree to not let anything pass your lips for twenty minutes after each meal. (Now it's Facebook/email time). Sadly, your stomach takes that long to realize it's full.

After waiting that long, ask yourself if you are still hungry before having any more food. You won't need anything else.

Your dietitian may have set you up to write a food diary. Make this part of your routine.

Try to make two slices of grain bread your daily limit.

Plan on having a good-sized lunch, then only a meagre meal in the evening, maybe only soup.

Hiding in your house are many unread recipe books. Pull one out and read the Fish chapter. You won't believe what you can learn here. How to select fish at the market, what steaming is, even poaching. It turns out that is something to do with *cooking* as well as catching trout on Mr.Gillmore's property.

Open the first seafood recipe and have a go. You cannot mess up fish. It's nature's own fast food. And before you disregard fish, remember how much you like fish'n'chips (with mushy peas if you are British). Then jump in.

What's turning up your nose right now is the smell of fish. And so it should. Nature's way of saying the fish is off. Fresh fish smells like the sea.

My first ever walk down Notting Hill's Portobello Road ended outside the fish monger's with me imploring my hosts who wanted to buy some NOT to go inside. *'There's something fishy in there!'* Problem is: when the whole shop stinks, it's hard to work out which dead animal is the offensive one.

Get friendly with a local fish monger who you can trust to teach you about fish. Mine works at my local supermarket and is opening the huge ice box when I arrive at the end of my thirty minute walk. (I don't count the ten minute walk back from the shops laden with shopping, that's weight training.)

One day I met his boss, the small chain's fish buyer. He starts work at three every morning in the city's fish market, buying the fish off the skippers. His selections are cleaned and filleted, then dispatched to the shops. My guy knows that he will be seeing me every day or so, and delights when I ask: *'Any dead fish?'* It attracts the attention of the other patrons. Knowing that I will be back to complain, he never steers me wrong. He also has the courage to shake his head if my favorite, sole, is missing from today's catch, or he is not happy with the quality. He knows that I have frozen a few days' supply in my fridge.

After a bit of fun in the kitchen (and two disasters) there is a possibility that you will learn to love fish with vegetables. The aircrew lifestyle means that, often, you can make a huge lunch at home while nine-to-fivers have to make do with tuna sandwiches. With a non-creamy vegetable soups after 4 p.m. the weight will start falling off after about ten days.

As your weight reduces the fat in your neck will vanish, leading to less (and even no) snoring, and may reduce problems you have with sleep apnea. You will also start sleeping seven to eight hours, which causes the weight to reduce further.

If you are seriously interested in dropping the weight further, by cutting back on processed foods, try doing this:

1) Go to your favorite hamburger chain and order the biggest, greasiest, fat-laden burger. Get a table and eat it slowly. Savor every mouthful.

2) Go home and watch the movie "FOOD INC." (It's on YouTube.) After seeing the documentary you will probably never eat processed meat ever again, which will be great for your figure.

The concept of being a vegetarian scared the life out of me, until I realized that my weekend breakfast of:

- juice,
- cereal,
- yogurt,
- two poached eggs balanced on sliced Roma

tomatoes, on top of avocado smashed into toast,
- Tea with milk and sugar,

was actually a vegetarian meal in itself.

It's possible to live happily ever-after eating grains, fruit, fish and vegetables while surviving on Laughter and Sex. But life may be enhanced if you treat yourself to a delicious restaurant-cooked grass-fed steak a few times a month.

Regular sex is healthy, say the experts. The editor of preventdisease.com[83] (well worth a browse) suggests that regular sex helps you:

- de-stress
- is a great form of exercise
- lowers high blood pressure
- builds your immunity
- makes you look younger
- is good for your heart
- provides pain relief
- builds trust and intimacy
- lessens your chances of contracting cancer
- builds stronger pelvic muscles
- protects your prostate (if you have one)
- provides regular periods (if you don't)
- prevents erectile dysfunction
- lengthens your life
- makes your semen healthier

I include all this, mainly as sales material for all young men who need help working on their pitch. After reading that, it appears to be the ultimate wonder drug. In reality, sex induces sleep in men after ejaculation and in women if you've been doing it right.

For men, there is evidence that you can't trick your body. While you can *induce* sleep with masturbation, the health effects benefitting prostate, heart, blood pressure and longevity can only be obtained by the sex act with a real person. Sorry guys.

If you need to sleep you know what to do.

And if sex isn't in your life then I am sure you can add a little chocolate.

RECAPPING:

- There is a direct correlation between weight and sleep quality.

- If you are overweight, your family and friends might not tell you.

- Being overweight can increase problems with snoring, sleep apnea and back pain.

- The airline industry, rightly or wrongly, promotes a below-weight, to normal-weight image.

- Some airlines are targeting overweight employees: "Lose it or leave."

- If you decide to get rid of the weight, get help from professionals.

- Build up a knowledge base by reading:

  "Love, Laugh, and Eat:
  And Other Secrets of Longevity from the
  Healthiest People on Earth"
  by Dr. John Tickell.

  "The China Study"
  by Campbell, Schurman and Campbell.

  "The Blue Zones"
  by Dan Buettner.

- Eat healthy food, no more than 2,000 calories a day and drink lots of water. This is not a diet, it is a lifestyle change.

- Embark on a daily exercise program.

- Sex is healthy (if you are doing it right).

- Sex induces sleep.

From the Logbook

My latest airline (the seventh) is paranoid about weight gain. They are fixated with Body Mass Index (B.M.I.) which gets the weight-training junkies in trouble because muscle is more dense than fat. Every year, prior to my aviation medical, I embark on a two-week weight-loss program to ensure that I tip the scales at the same weight I was the day they employed me. Chicken noodle soup for lunch and dinner.

I am ready to reply, if they say that I am too fat: *'Well you shouldn't have employed me - should you?'*

They say that regular sex makes you look ten years younger. I was told that about cycling. I know what I'd much rather do on a cold winter morning.

Update

In July 2015 Singapore's CEO, Goh Choon Phong, told FlightGlobal.com[84] that Singapore Girl will remain front and center as the face of the airline:

'Subtle changes have taken place with the Singapore Girl," he says. *"Recently the make-up was changed and we do update her so that she is more contemporary, but the grace and service culture she represents is absolutely something we want to preserve. This will continue.'*

Part Two

Things you have to do to sleep better

Sleep Preparation

Flight Preparation

The law requires that:

"… Flight crew members are adequately rested at the beginning of each Flying Duty Period …"

To that end, arriving at the aircraft fatigued is against the law, not to mention stupid. This unpredictable industry may require you to perform a passenger evacuation within minutes of pushing-back. And when was the last time you did one of those for real?

Forget that your passengers are expecting a standard of safety and professionalism from you, there is a real chance that you could be in mortal danger. Your ability to think and act clearly may make the difference between an exciting story or painful, excruciating injuries, a completely changed future, or even death.

We're kidding right? Sadly no. Victims of air crashes and incidents will tell you that they didn't think they'd be having an incident that day either. An unnerving percentage of crashes occur during the first flight of the day. Having been interviewed by safety investigators after an incident (it was only an engine shutdown and diversion) it was enlightening to see how they do their job. They were interested in running their process as, thankfully, they had little practical experience.

Question One:

'Tell us about what you ate in the day before the incident'.

Question Two:

'How much sleep did you get the day before the incident, and the day before that?'

Flying around tired is the equivalent of flying around drunk, and we know how funny they are about that. If you want to make a long-term career out of this profession, you must get to grips with this concept:

"The best way to get rest before the flight is by taking control of your life and ensuring a large slab of preflight sleep".

Sleep Early

Going to bed for a few hours before a flight is rarely successful; you need about five or six hours. Eight if you can get them. The reason you have had problems sleeping before duty periods before is that you have not slept *early* enough. By grabbing only a few hours, your subconscious mind spends most of its time worried that you will sleep through the alarm. This means you never get into that deep REM sleep which detoxifies your body, solves problems, loses weight, and makes you look nice.

Try sleeping for eight full hours. With enough alarm clocks set to wake a football team billeted in different suburbs, your brain *knows* that there is *no chance* you will sleep-in and will allow you to have a deep sleep. Ideally you will wake up naturally after about six or seven hours, without hearing even one hideous alarm clock. That's shift-worker bliss. In fact, you may find that with good management you only wake up to an alarm clock a few times a month. Something the nine-to-fivers in your life could only dream about.

Before an evening sign-on for a night flight, you have to manage your *previous* day's sleep so that you get to bed early, and naturally wake up early. Then embark on early exercise, either in the gym or a long walk, which will make it easier to sleep during the afternoon.

Hibernate

Tell your family and friends that you will not be available for the time prior to your duty. We already blocked it off in our roster (*see the "Rosters & Diaries" chapter*) as "Sleep Time" which includes an eight hour block plus the time to get ready, plus the time to get to the airport. We are talking about ten to eleven hours before your duty period starts.

Your friends and family must be aware that you are *uncontactable* during this rest phase. They don't contact you when you are flying in the sky and they must *not* contact you when you are resting before the flight. Accepting this is the key to a successful career in the airline business. Let everybody know that you will not be available from a specific time. Do not bend. Even if you are awake and see their messages, do not respond. 90% of this is training others. And, make no mistake, like a puddle-making puppy, they can be trained. But you need self-discipline.

Securing this time takes some doing; you even have to learn to lie about it. It's easier for single people because you can lie without getting caught out, but it's tough for married people and very tough for people with children. You need a supportive partner, preferably one who understands the type of shift-work you do. And unless they have done it, they never really get it. It's why cabin crew marry pilots and nurses marry doctors. Why air traffic controllers, immigration, customs and police marry their own. You need to know that someone else will pick up the kids from school and keep them quietly playing at the other end of the house. Someone will protect your sleep fiercely. There are few divorces amongst aviation couples who get this principle. It's a team effort.

Next you have to trick your body into believing that it is time to sleep. Late in the morning draw the blinds and curtains, turn on lights, have a main meal as if it is evening. Watch a movie or TV program that you normally would watch at night. This is ideal if you have a boxed set DVDs of a TV program you like, or have the ability on your television to record programs.

Stick a note on your door which says "Do Not Disturb."

Unplug the land line and turn your mobile phone onto flight mode. If you turn it off completely the alarm may not work. You may wish to write a note reminding yourself that the phones are off, and place it where you will see it.

Ensure that everything is done. Your uniform is ready.

If you are doing a layover have your suitcase almost ready to close.

Go online to weatherunderground.com[85] and check out the weather conditions at your destination to help you pack appropriately. Don't be one of those crew members who arrives in a destination and says:

'Oh, I didn't pack any clothes!'

You want to explore destinations, take advantage of

good weather, or just get exercise. By packing for the conditions you are not going to be tied to your hotel room which, you guessed it, leads to sleeping inappropriately. There is also your future grandchildren to think of. I have done many flights to Paris and can sadly state that a percentage crew have never left the hotel, which is close to the airport. Imagine the conversation when your grandchildren say:

'Wow, grandma, you are so cool! You were an international flight attendant! What was Paris like?'

'I dunno, I never left the hotel...'

Once you get to your destination you can dress for the conditions and go out to explore the world, which is why you took this job. This will get you sufficiently tired if you can push through the exhaustion from the previous flight, stay awake as long as you can, and be ready to sleep.

If crashing when you arrive is *inappropriate*, what is *appropriate* sleep? Simple. You have already planned your sleep prior to your next flight when you got your roster at the beginning of the month. You know you have to get eight hours sleep before the next duty period, so work backwards from that. If you did not sleep well prior to the outbound flight grab two or three hours' sleep but set multiple alarms so that you wake up and enjoy the local lunchtime and afternoon if you can. An incentive is to make lunch or early dinner dates with friends who live in that city.

With good planning, these are the only alarms that will wake you up all month. You must get out and about, which means having the correct clothing.

Packing

You are packed ready to go. Or are you?

Packing is the easiest thing on the earth for a

seasoned airline professional. Our friends and relatives cannot believe how good we are at this. But those of us new to the profession may need a quick lesson:

"To pack quickly, have a shower."

When you come out of the shower dry yourself and start putting on clothes. For each article of clothing that you put on, grab articles to pack. Undies? How many will you need? Three? Add one extra pair in case of an aircraft breakdown. Then put them on the bed.

Socks? How many will you need? Add an extra pair, put them on the bed.

Shirts? And so on, don't forget shoes.

Now your bed is covered with all the clothes that you will need to pack.

Fold or roll? Shirts are folded and slid into stiff plastic bags so that they retain their ironed-shape. This way they will look great once put on a hanger for eight hours, maybe only needing a quick touch-up. Every shoe is wrapped in a shopping plastic bag, each one stuffed with socks, undies or a belt to save space. Skivvies, pants, sweaters, and t-shirts benefit from being rolled, or cleverly folded.

There are some great YouTube videos on packing suitcases. The most impressive is great if you are moving houses, but aircrew have to live out of their suitcases since we never know if bed bugs will be an issue.

A separate bag is needed for phone chargers, USB cables, and the electronic plugs required for various destinations. If you do not know which plug to take, go on the internet and search the country name plus the words "electrical plugs." You will find a long list of electrical plugs and the requirements. Most airline crew have electrical plugs that cater for all locations.

How about on the inside of your suitcase lid you stick a post-it note asking yourself:

'Do I need that big jacket?'

This will act as a mental reminder before you close your suitcase. When going to cold destinations we often remember to dress appropriately but then forget to take our big jacket.

You are now packed, except for your wet-pack/makeup. Your uniform is ready and now to relax your brain by having a chamomile tea or hot chocolate.

Check your roster for changes and if on a layover, check the arrival time of your incoming flight. It's not worth sleeping now if the only plane you can operate is ten hours late. Perform a Google[86] search. Put in your company's flight number and press enter.

For American Airlines flight 109, enter: AA109

For Qantas flight 1, enter: QF1

For Etihad flight 406, enter: EY406

This gives you the status of that inbound flight showing you if it took off on time and showing the estimated time of arrival. Knowing that there has been no change to your hotel departure time means that you can sleep heavily without your subconscious asking the question every few minutes:

'What time do I have to wake up?'

Sleep early, sleep heavily ... wake up naturally.

RECAPPING:

- The best way to get rest before the flight is by taking control of your life and ensuring a large slab of pre-flight sleep.

- Block off at least eight hours before you need to wake.

- Be UNcontactable to everyone during your blocked-off sleep time.

- Pack before you sleep.

- Check your inbound flight and roster before you sleep.

- Sleep early, sleep heavily and wake up naturally.

From the Logbook

Discovering the principle of quarantining sleep time before a duty led to my contacting my widowed mother more often. Rather than worry that she needed anything, or having my subconscious nagging me while I tried to sleep:

'Waargh! The phone is off. What if your mother needs you?'

I found it easier to ring her and say hello before going to sleep. It made me feel better and had an added side-effect when I heard her remark to someone:

'The Captain* makes me feel that <u>every</u> day is Mother's Day!'

Little did she know, I was just trying to sleep better.

---

* *She used my real name.*

At Nairobi, Kenya the crew of a freighter did not check the status of inbound flight. They went downstairs, checked out of the hotel, jumped in the transport and went to the airport. After officially signing-on they found themselves standing at the freight terminal, astounded to find their plane was not only invisible, but was hours from arrival.

Their duty was to fly to Amsterdam and by the time their plane arrived they would have exceeded the roster duty time limits. They had to go back to the hotel and take minimum rest while their plane arrived and sat dormant before they resumed their flight to Amsterdam. This delayed their arrival into Amsterdam and that of the cargo, tons of freshly-cut flowers destined for international markets.

A quick check on Google or the company's website before going to sleep may have alerted them to ring operations, work out that someone had forgotten to notify them, change the hotel departure time and get the flowers to the destination as fast as possible.

Room Preparation

Black Out The Room

To get sleep when you want, the room must be completely blacked-out. At home this includes having a blackout blind covered with a blackout curtain and making sure that no light escapes into your room. When negotiating the deal with the blind/curtain supplier, make payment dependent on a successful outcome which can be done by checking the result during daytime.

Take a few clothes pegs with you in your suitcase and use them to secure the gap where hotel curtains meet. At the extreme edges of the curtains it is sometimes necessary to use pillows, cushions, bathroom towels, the standard lamp or other furniture to contrive a means of holding the curtain flat against the wall so that no light escapes into the room. The bedspread (counterpane) is then stuffed along the floor to seal the gap under the curtains. To make sure that all light from under the main hotel room door is blocked, a bath mat, towel or dressing-gown helps to close off the light and fill what is often a huge gap. It also helps minimize noise sneaking in to disrupt your sleep and also keeps out smoke. Your mission is to block every light source, especially blue light.

From the bed your eyes will be attracted to power supply light on the television. Some of the stiff cardboard cards, maybe the room service menu, or face washer, can be put in front of the red LED light. The digital alarm clock should be turned away from the bed and also covered to stop light from reflecting. When the room is pitch dark you can sleep properly. If there is any, repeat *any*, light approaching your eyes even when asleep your sleep will not be as sound.

Empty Your Brain

Place a note pad and pencil beside your bed. Before you go to sleep, or as you are trying to sleep you will remind yourself of a friend's birthday, you have to email somebody, to buy something, or pay a bill. Write these down.

Don't Go To Bed Angry

Note down anything that is clamming-up your brain. If you need a question answered write it down. The task of writing it down can sometimes spur your subconscious into solving the problem when you are sleeping.

Use a Pencil

"Creative waking" means that you can write down your thoughts while curled up in bed at any angle without your pen failing to write.

Read a Book

Read a book, any book, preferably one that is interesting enough to keep your attention but boring enough so that you can fall asleep while reading it. The light shining onto the pages from the overhead reading light in the fully darkened room reflects up into your eyes and helps make you drowsy. If you are using an iPad as your eReader, reverse the text so it is a black page with dark grey text; then turn the brightness right down.

Blue Light

Studies have shown that short-wave, blue light, associated with mobile phones, televisions, iPads, computers, and some models of backlit eReaders can stop you falling asleep. Reading only real books (or Kindles) in the last hour before bed (some say three hours) can help. Or you can get special globes and glasses from lowbluelights.com[87].

Sex or Sleep Only

Make a rule with yourself that your bed and bedroom is for sleeping and sex only. Lying in bed reading for hours, using your iPod or phone, watching television or movies, tricks your brain into believing that the bed is for other activities. If you can train your brain to associate bed with sleep or sex and nothing else, then it makes it easier to fall asleep (or have sex!) when you are in bed.

Cool Temperature

It's healthy to make the room temperature fairly cool allowing you to snuggle up in bed and sleep. About 18°C (65F) is ideal. As you sleep, your body temperature heats the bed and the room so it is best to start off with cool temperature.

Television

Despite what people think, the truth is that *the devil lives in television*. And he takes your soul by endlessly playing that Sky News theme. There is something different between reading books and watching television when it comes to helping people sleep. TV plays tricks with your brain and messes with the sleep initiation sequence.

During a layover, only turn on the television for a specific program you have planned to watch. Channel surfing is dangerous. Ideally, never turn on a television in a hotel room during a layover. Anyone who has been in this industry for any length of the time will agree with me:

> "No pilot or cabin crew has ever seen a full movie
> from start to finish during a layover."

We have all seen the beginnings and endings, but a full movie? Rarely. Ask them to recall what they have seen. Chances are their brain was mush and they didn't get the full movie experience. That is, except for *"The Silence of the Lambs."* I saw that in a hotel room in Wagga Wagga and it stopped me sleeping for days afterwards. The TV stays off.

Ear Plugs

Obtain some earplugs with the maximum Noise Reduction Rating (NRR) of 32 decibels, the industrial strength foam plugs available from pharmacies. It is important to train yourself to use the earplugs over about a week to mask extraneous noise while you sleep so you can have confidence before you try using them on a layover or before a night flight.

There is a correct way to insert them, compressing and rolling them, using your saliva to make a seal, then insert and hold them in position for ten seconds until the foam expands. You need to gain confidence that you can still hear your alarm clocks even though you are wearing earplugs. Eventually you will become proficient at sleeping while using earplugs and will choose to use them all the time. They are fantastic when going on holidays and finding that there is a three-year-old in the motel room next door. Turn up the Absolute Sleep Music (or white noise soundscape) making it loud enough hear, even with the earplugs. This should mask nearly all of the extraneous noise.

Sleeping Masks

There are various types of sleep mask, often handed out by airlines. A comfortable silk version, from an online seller Hibermate.com[88], incorporates ear muffs together with a sleep mask. These are fantastic for use in-aircraft as a passenger, but I find them too hot to use in crew rest or bed. It also takes a while to get used to sleeping using a sleep mask. Start tonight.

Pillows

Pillows are the bane of every a crew member. I have met crew who take their favorite pillow with them whenever they go on layover. Grab all the pillows when you get in the room, including the one or two in the top of the wardrobe, and choose your favorites. Don't be timid. Jammed up against our backs, to be used as something to hug, or to block cracks of light from invading the room. They are all to be used. Twisted, bent, misshapen, pounded; we do all sorts of things to pillows to get adequate rest and you should too.

The mark of a good hotel is the quality of their pillows and their offer to bring firm pillows, when needed. Ring room service.

Pajamas

People who never wear pajamas at home may choose to when on the road. The concept of bed bugs and mites make you think that it is better to be completely covered. That includes socks. Another reason for using pajamas during layovers in hotel rooms is that you find there are wayward air-conditioning breezes. Such a gale hitting the back of your neck at the wrong angle can make sleep difficult. Pajamas can help.

Sleep Socks

While I have never explored using *sleep gloves,* if your toes and fingertips get cold I can report that big fluffy socks can help after allowing the room temperature to be lowered. This makes it easier to get to sleep.

Tiger Balm Eucalyptus

Try a Tiger Balm Eucalyptus foot rub before you go to sleep then put on warm fluffy socks. This can sometimes prove relaxing when you have a cold. Try it to aid sleeping.

Alarm Clocks

While your brain is worried about getting to sleep, and then worried about waking up in time for your flight, you will never get into deep REM sleep. Without a deep sleep your body does not restore itself as designed. The way to achieve deep sleep is to have a number of alarm clocks ranging in intensity from a favorite song to the most horrid electronic beeping imaginable.

The wake up sequence begins with the iPad with Absolute Sleep Music (or equivalent) providing the heavy rains or white noise, and when the musical alarm starts (a favored song), it is enough to wake you up. A few minutes later your telephone which was set to flight mode is set to start up a loud, but soothing, wake-up alarm.

At your planned wake up time, your iPod Touch has an alarm which is loud and persistent. Try using "sonar" as the alarm tone, and see if you can sleep through it. Five minutes later the last resort is the trusted battery-operated alarm clock with the hideous electronic beeping alarm that can (and will) wake people in the room three doors down. As soon as the first alarm goes, turn on the lights and get out of bed. Never remain in bed and never hit a snooze button.

Pets

No pets in the bedroom when you are sleeping. A pet in the bedroom means the door is open, allowing them to come and go, and light to enter which goes against the rules of sleeping.

Back Pain

Thousands of airline pilots share their careers with debilitating back pain. Curled up sleeping in the same position can exacerbate back pain, especially after hours sitting in cockpit seats.

Finding a good sleeping position is important. Some Tiger Balm rubbed in the small of your back prior to sleeping may help. If it is a real muscle problem the heat will expand the nerve sheath and cause pain. If this is the case ice is needed, which contracts the nerve, or an anti-inflammatory like Voltaren or its safer sister, faster-acting Cataflam. Your doctor will have the right idea.

Physiotherapists recommend sleeping with a pillow jammed between your knees to lay your spine in the perfect position. Good luck trying to sleep in this manner. I am yet to find anyone who sleeps this way (besides the Editor of this book).

There are exercises which, if done every day, strengthen the core muscles which help hold your vertebrae in the correct position. The Mayo Clinic's website has examples complete with photos to ensure you understand the correct positions[89].

Losing weight off your front also reduces back pain. But nothing beats a visit to a physiotherapist. It pays to have a professional take a look at your gait and devise some exercises specifically targeting your issues.

RECAPPING:

- **Black out the room.**
- **Empty your brain with pencil and paper.**
- **Don't go to bed angry.**
- **Read a book.**
- **Sex or Sleep Only.**
- **Cool the room down.**
- **Turn off the television.**
- **Learn to use ear plugs.**
- **And sleep masks.**
- **There are no rules about pillows. Use as many as you need.**
- **Pajamas and sleep socks may make you feel more comfortable in hotels.**
- **Tiger Balm your feet for a relaxing sleep.**
- **No pets.**
- **If you suffer back pain, get it sorted.**

From the Logbook

'In order to fall asleep, you have to *pretend* to be asleep'
> *- (Internet quote by a comedian which started in 2013. Am yet to find the author)*

Twice a year I was suffering debilitating lower back pain, or Sciatica. My doctor prescribed an M.R.I. scan to see what was going on.

When I shared the images with a physiotherapist, he demanded to know who had diagnosed me with Sciatica. Crestfallen, I sheepishly said:

'*Um … me!*'

He rolled his young eyes and muttered:

'*Doctor Bloody Google again. This is not sciatica!*'

Then proceeded to show me pictures of my lower discs which were the problem.

A few balancing exercises on the fit ball, planking, a few yoga moves and a change to my treadmill sessions was all that was needed.

'*Try using the treadmill on the flat. People use it on a grade which puts pressure on the two discs in question*'

The result: no more "sciatica." I would have seen him a few years earlier, *but he was still in kindergarten.*

The Bed & Position

The Bed

You know it when you find it. The perfect mattress. Aircrew are lucky because we get to sample at least thirty beds a year. When you find one, have a look at the label and write down the name and model. Armed with the details of your ideal sleeping partner, race into a bed shop and do a deal. They'll be shocked at how fast they can rack up a sale that you can make it conditional that they deliver the new one, fully install it and take away the old bed. I have even made a deal over the phone, the fastest sale they've ever made.

Experts say that a bed only lasts five years, but you can extend that to ten by turning the mattress over, then spinning it around every three months. They say you should sleep on the other side of hotel beds to the telephone, to avoid where hundreds of travelling salesmens' bums have sat as they made their calls. But I believe most smart hotels rotate their mattresses regularly to extend their lives. Besides, these days the smart salesman would sit at the desk, computer open, updating their customer relationship management program as they talk on the phone.

Bedding

100% cotton sheets provide you with a better sleep than poly/cotton (which are much cheaper), and while your mother will tell you that a high thread count Egyptian cotton sheets are the only way to go, it is sadly no longer true. Thread count means the number of fibers per square inch and 1,000 used to be gold standard.

Sadly since our moms' day the nefarious manufacturers have been blending and twisting lesser quality fibers to achieve the same result. Your 1,000 thread count sheet may be only 250 thread four-ply with inferior cotton strands. In that case a real 180 thread strand pure cotton sheet may last you longer. In this throwaway age you are better off going for a lower thread count cotton over any type of poly/cotton.

Duvets/doonas or blankets? Anyone who has been forced to spend a night in a hotel in France during a heatwave in April knows the answer: sheets and blankets. How is it that an entire country has hotels with only two settings on the air-conditioning: summer and winter?

The control box in the room has no effect. Ringing down to the reception to plead for the engineer to come and fix my air conditioner (it was 26C/79F outside and 30C/86F inside) I was told in no uncertain terms: *'Eet ees not May yet.'* Apparently May 1st is the day they flick a big switch from winter to summer. A decade later in another French city, same story.

Duvets are often filled with polyester fiber, not down, and heat control can be impossible. Cotton blankets for warm climates and pure wool blankets in colder places allow you to achieve perfect temperature control. Natural fibers are better in fires. Soaked in water they can save your life.

Bed Placement

Feng shui, the ancient Chinese concept of human interaction with the elements, has a number of rules, known by expensive interior decorators. If you apply the elements, life is grand and you become healthy and successful. You will sleep better surrounded by curved lines, no sharp edges, a bed against a solid wall with a night table on each side with the bed placed in a way that you can see the door, but not facing it, with effective airflow from both sides and underneath the bed, and under a non-sloping ceiling with no fan or chandelier above.

If a mirror faces the bed you can expect to be dead by morning.

Much of this makes sense. Ask anyone who has slept in a cheap hotel with a door at the foot of their bed. Hall light flooding under the door makes sleep hard to obtain. But, for me, feng shui is all in the mind.

As it should be.

It makes sense that your sleep is uninterrupted by feelings of insecurity. If you are in control of designing your bedroom then do whatever it takes to make your bedroom feel good to you. Everyone should feel safe and snug when they sleep.

The internet's feng shui masters lost me when they suggested you shouldn't have a television in the room, as television wasn't invented in ancient China.

No doubt, the power of the mind is limitless, and positive thoughts can't hurt before trying to sleep.

RECAPPING:

- Do you own research from sleeping around, and find the make and model of your ideal bed.

- Then buy it.

- Turn the mattress over and/or rotate it every season.

- Buy a new one every five to ten years.

- Hotel mattresses: use the opposite side to where peoples' bums sit if it makes you feel better.

- Buy cotton and wool bedding which allows you to control the temperature of your sleeping experience. Especially in a fire.

- Adopt Feng shui bed placement, or face your head north, east, south or west if it makes you feel better. But is it a reason to knock down the wall?

Self-Hypnosis & Relaxation Techniques

If you have ever tried relaxing with a self-meditation or hypnosis program you will have fixed opinions. It either works or it doesn't. Having a voice tell you what to do works if you like the voice. Often when you're about to sleep they ring a gong as if they are some kind of an ashram policeman demanding that you relax. Then you are instantly wide awake and annoyed.

Good luck finding the correct audiobook recording; there are hundreds to choose from. Here's hoping that you find the ideal voice and pace for you. For me, often these practitioners sound like salesmen trying to flog something and two of them are personal friends which doesn't work as I keep seeing their faces.

For those of us who don't respond to the audio relaxation sessions, there are techniques that can be done in your sleeping position or in the 'traditional way' on your back. For a start, wear loose-fitting clothing, be warm, and lie on a firm surface with pillows or cushions propping you up. A pillow under your knees may feel more comfortable.

Grab enough of the bedclothes at the bottom of the bed so that they loosely cover your feet which, for the exercise, will be splayed outwards. There is nothing as distracting as tight bedclothes putting pressure on your toes. Well, there is, I suppose; a particularly frisky monkey jumping on the bed would get your full and undivided attention, but stick with me here.

Having made yourself comfortable in a dark room with no distractions, concentrate on relaxing your body and trying to sink into the bed. Unclench your jaw, relax and soften your face muscles and realize how different it feels. Adopt a breathing pattern that fits with the mood; try different types until one feels right. Are you breathing with your nose or only through your mouth?

Some people purposefully try to empty their minds with a "mantra" or sound as they breathe out. 'Ommmm' was a popular meditative sound of the 1960s and 70s. The vibrations in your lips and skull block out other noise. With heavy rain or white noise going, maybe you don't need a mantra.

As thoughts flood your brain, 'Did I lock the front door?', 'I have to pay my car registration this week' ... recognize the thought, then move it off to the left or right and know you will recall it tomorrow. Persistent thoughts obviously need your attention; write them down on the pad next to your bed and start the relaxation exercise again. With practice you can see a thought coming, nod to it and send it on its way.

When you are ready, take three deep breaths. Before we start, are you breathing correctly?

An exercise taught at radio announcing/acting school to use the diaphragm for better breathing and speech production utilizes an upturned kitchen broom. Wedge the end of the long handle between the floor and wall and place the broom head against the chest (use a clean one), lean into it and learn to breathe using the diaphragm. The chest should remain still as you breathe in. The tummy goes in and out. To empty the lungs the tummy comes in, with the diaphragm pushing the air up and out.

Read copy or sing and notice the difference and control.

The lungs can be filled, and filled and filled. Some students discover that they have been breathing incorrectly. Others find that they have never really filled their lungs before, only ever breathing off the top of their lungs. This is rare in pilots who have had to pass the lung volume test for their medicals, but for cabin crew it helps them to understand why they have been suffering the mild effects of hypoxia for their entire airborne lives.

When you find a person having a panic attack they are breathing off the top off their lungs and getting a CO_2 buildup. Getting them to focus on breathing correctly gets them under control.

Being able to deep breathe in this manner, filling to capacity then holding the breath momentarily, then expelling until there is nothing left. And holding that pose for a few seconds before repeating the cycle three times in a row oxygenates the lungs. Try it at least once a waking hour and often during exercise. With a few sips of water, it is an effective inflight pick-me-up.

Having taken three deep breaths, in your relaxation pose, scrunch up all your muscles, ball your fists, screw up your toes, your eyes, your mouth and nose; hold a few seconds, then release. Notice the difference between being scrunched-up and tense, then going completely soft and sinking into the bed.

Fully relax, then slowly survey your body from the toes up your legs, your bottom, back, up to your neck and face including your arms and fingers. Scrunch up and tense every muscle in turn, hold, then release. Hold each pose for about five to ten seconds.

When you get to your face scrunch up your eyes, then open them as wide as possible, purse your lips, then open your mouth as wide as possible in a yawn. *(That's why we do this in a dark room so you don't scare the kiddies.)*

Then lie in a relaxed state for ten minutes.

Some practitioners recommend getting up and shaking out your limbs noting how refreshed you are. I prefer to roll over on my side and sleep. Which is the name of the game.

RECAPPING:
- **Try guided relaxation exercises; if one works for you, use it.**
- **If you find them annoying, use the principles and try self-relaxation.**
- **Learn to breathe properly using the diaphragm. Chest remains still, tummy gets fat as your breathe in. Tummy gets skinny as you breathe out.**
- **Settle into a relaxed pose in a dark room.**
- **Take a deep breath, then even more, and even more and hold it a few seconds before breathing out. Then holding that too.**
- **Repeat three times.**

- **Scrunch up all your muscles at once, hold for five seconds and release.**
- **Starting at your toes, visualize each muscle group and scrunch and release all the way up your body. Toes, feet, legs, bottom, fingers, hands arms, shoulders, torso, neck and face.**
- **Relax, then sleep.**

From the Logbook

After one yoga class some people stayed on for a guided relaxation session. The Type A's all jumped up and raced off as soon as the class was finished while the rest of us lay around like sun-baking sea lions. Three quarters of the way through the session a tiny old lady started snoring like a drunken sailor.

Trying not to laugh is infectious. Before long the entire class disintegrated into laughter and had to be abandoned to the tea room.

The little old lady slept on.

Pre-Sleep Affirmations

No-one can tell if there is a god, but there is evidence in nearly every culture that humans benefit from pre-sleep talking to:

- Allah
- God
- Dead relatives
- Spiritual guides
- Their own brains (in the form of visualizations and affirmations)

Be it a cleansing of the soul, clearing the decks for sleep, visualizing success, programing your subconscious or something greater than all of us; you'd be hard-pressed to say it doesn't work.

Ask a top-level sportsperson or other type of high achiever. Self-talk and "seeing" success are all a part of preparation. Few pilots would enter a simulator for their license renewal without having first sat quietly and visualized going through a perfect performance. In fact the "6Ps" are well-known in the industry:

"Perfect Preparation Prevents
Piss Poor Performance."

We were led to believe that it was an Air Force saying, but it probably dates back to before planes were flying.

A wise man once suggested that before sleep you should review the day and the positive things you did for three people that:

(a) they did not know about, or

(b) they knew about but no-one else does,

(and that you will keep secret).

While you are about it you can ask for the answers to the questions you posed on your pad as you were emptying your brain before sleep.

Then tell your brain what time it is now and when you would like to wake up. Some people are good at this and always wake up a minute before their alarm clock.

Finally, ask The Universe / God / Allah / Spiritual Guides / Dead Relatives for a great night's sleep and for them to watch over you.

With practice you'll get to sleep faster, and sleep sounder. Your subconscious will beaver away at the problems all night and provide answers in the morning.

RECAPPING:

- **People report that pre-sleep affirmations, visualizations work.**

- **Before you sleep, review the positive effect you have made on three peoples' lives that day.**

- **Train your brain to wake yourself up at the time you would like.**

- **Ask whoever it is that you are comfortable with for a good nights' sleep. It may work.**

From the Logbook

As explained at the end of the Alcohol chapter, three rooms at the Canberra Hyatt hotel are almost underground. Someone told the Cabin Crew that they were haunted and their union arranged that they never had to stay in them. The three rooms became the province of the Captain, First Officer and Flight Engineer of the last nightly airplane into Canberra, a Boeing 727.

When arriving in the room, every time, I said hello to the ghosts and thanked them for having me in their room.

I explained that I was tired and needed to sleep, and would they mind not bothering me during the night?

They never did.

Waking-Up

As stated before, if you can mentally train yourself to wake up at the same time every day you can often beat the alarm clock. Before you go to bed, say the time out loud and the time you would like to wake up. Noticing it or silently thinking about it does not seem to be as successful. The first time you wake up without the alarm clock, only to be given a nasty shock seconds later as the alarm activates you will think it a coincidence. After the third time you will start to think it is a little freaky.

No-one knows how smart your brain is.

However, few aircrew have the luxury of a regular wake-up time.

There is something wrong about waking up unnaturally. From an early age we should train our brains to believe that an alarm clock wake-up is unnatural. Waking up *without* the alarm clock is bliss. It's why people retire from work or go on annual leave. By planning your roster for the month and scheduling sleep, you will find that you will sleep longer before night flights and wake up without alarm clocks.

Do not press the snooze button. Treat it as if it is connected to live electricity.

Get straight out of bed. Try to decipher what you wrote on the bedside pad during the night and think about questions from the previous night. Chances are the answers are now clear in your mind. Write them down. Don't trust your memory.

Make your bed. This is a trick the military have developed. It stops you going back to sleep and prevents creepy crawlies getting in. You give your subconscious a sense of achievement, a portent for the rest of the day. It looks good, which enhances your pride. And it gives you something inviting to come back to when you arrive home tired. *(You don't have to do this if you wake up in a hotel.)*

If you are trying to lose weight (see the weight chapter) then weigh yourself, check your blood pressure, fill in your figures in your sleep diary.

Glance at your schedule and decide your day's goals as you do your stretches.

Plan your fitness, straight away or later?

The more you can develop a routine for sleeping and waking, the easier life becomes for the career pilot or cabin crew. You can shift the timings, but your body will thank you and you will feel more in control. Feeling in control when some unnamed person in an office is pulling the strings of your life a month in advance is what's needed to turn this job into a long-term career.

RECAPPING:

- Before you go to bed, say the time out loud and the time you would like to wake up.
- When you wake up, never press an alarm's snooze button.
- Get straight out of bed.
- Look at the pad beside your bed. If you had pondered a question the night before, do you have an answer? If so, write it down your immediate reaction.
- Make your bed.
- If you are trying to lose weight, or track blood pressure etc., fill in your diary and sleep diary now.
- Check out your diary and think about your day's goals while doing stretches.
- Plan your fitness.
- Developing a routine will help you feel that you have more control over your life even when it's determined by a crew roster.
- The more comfortable with your life, the better you sleep.

From the Logbook

My idea of the ultimate month is managing to wake up naturally, that is, without an alarm clock, on all occasions except for the days I arrive at a layover destination in the early morning.

On such a day I will sleep for only a few hours using the alarm to rouse me, before going for a long lunch. I choose ninety minutes if possible, so I am waking up at the end of a sleep cycle. With completely blacked-out hotel rooms, I will wake at this time with no idea of where I am. Sometimes it is unnerving when there is a wall in the wrong place.

There are stories of crew who have walked out in the hallway, thinking they were going to the bathroom, only to realize their mistake upon hearing the door click behind them. Embarrassing if you sleep naked. Luckily most hotels have a house phone near the elevator.

[Except one particular hotel in Melbourne: the *Rockman's Regency*. The night after a Christmas party, in the early 1980s, a famous visiting American radio correspondent had to go all the way down to the front desk to get a new key card; *without wearing a stitch*].

On the trips where you wake up after only 90 minutes sleep, even after a hot shower it's still possible to feel a little disorientated by the time you get to the restaurant. Be extremely careful crossing roads; tourists are often run over after forgetting that the traffic flow is the reverse of their home countries.

It's worth pushing through. The disorientation goes away, and being exposed to afternoon sunlight makes it easier to sleep the following night.

At Work

Mental Attitude

We have all worked with the "Sad Sack," the person who is complaining from the second we meet them. There is a reason why people call them "hard work." Everything is a problem: the company is trying to get them, the people they live with are disasters, their roster is worse than anyone else in the airline, they never sleep before a flight because there is always a work crew outside their bedroom window building a nuclear missile silo. And on and on. It never stops.

Not only do they bring everyone down, they make time stand still. A short flight becomes a long flight. A long flight becomes an ultra-long flight. An ultra-long flight becomes a never-ending nightmare. After a few hours you start considering that "Thou Shalt Not Kill" was written before this person arrived on the planet. It doesn't apply to them. Before the long-haul flight is half distance, murderous plans are hatched.

Don't be that person.

Instead, look in the mirror and smile at yourself. Say Hello. Thank your spiritual guides/gods/dead relatives/etc. for a great sleep and tell yourself, out loud, that you are going to have a great day. List the things that you are going to do well, being the best that you can be.

Agree with yourself that you are not going to bother others with negative talk, and try to ensure that if you can't say something nice about someone, you are not going to say anything. Plan to put yourself in other people's shoes before flying off the handle, and see things from their perspective. Recognize that, even though they are an absolute idiot who should not be allowed to handle hot objects, they have a family who love them, and next door neighbors who trust them enough to collect their mail and take out their garbage when they are on holidays. Children and small animals like them.

So watch and think before opening your mouth.

This smarmy stuff, the chapter about self-affirmations, and this one, actually works. Tell yourself you are feeling great and you will. No-one knows why.

Three American authors have done more than any others to promote self-belief, *Napoleon Hill* and *Dale Carnegie* and *Dr. Maxwell Maltz*. Their life stories are worth studying because every self-help book borrows their wisdom.

Napoleon Hill

Napoleon Hill reacted to a challenge by the rich industrialist, Andrew Carnegie, that he research why people were successful. Carnegie thought that the laws of physics, mathematics, and gravity must also have a parallel with human success. Why were some people were successful and others not?

After being introduced to Henry Ford by Carnegie, Hill then interviewed hundreds of successful people to arrive at his conclusions detailed in the massive *"The Laws of Success"* published in 1928. The more manageable *"Think and Grow Rich[90]"* was produced in 1937 and is still in print today. By 2011 it had sold more than seventy million copies.

He came up with the concept of *"mastermind,"* (what the advertising agencies and management gurus sprout as *"synergy"*) where two people working on an issue produce the results of three due to their bouncing ideas off each other. 1+1=3. Creatively, John Lennon and Paul McCartney are an example of mastermind in action. The method was employed by the U.S.President Franklin Delano Roosevelt in his formulation of the New Deal, the policy that dragged America out of the Great Depression. Hill supposedly wrote FDR's famous line:

'We have nothing to fear, but fear itself.'

Even though *"Think & Grow Rich"* made huge money, he had given his second wife (and probably co-author) the profits in a prenuptial agreement. After their divorce, he was left with nothing[91]. Hill went on to write another best seller and started Success Unlimited magazine.

Dale Carnagey/Carnegie

A Missouri farm boy who had worked multiple jobs before becoming a salesman, Dale Carnagey wanted to be on the circuit as a travelling tent lecturer, the tonight-show host of the time. To that end he ended up studying acting in New York. Broke and living at the Y.M.C.A., he convinced the manager to allow him to give a lecture to the other guests in return for 80% of the take. It was 1912. By 1914 he was giving courses on self-confidence and public speaking and making huge money.

After fighting in WWI he returned to the lecture and training business, and in 1922 changed the spelling of his name to benefit from the association with famous Andrew Carnegie who had died three years earlier. He hired and gave lectures in Carnegie Hall to further blur the association.

By the pit of the depression he was delivering a course which became the book *"How to Win Friends and Influence People*[92]*."* Today it is still in print and has sold more than fifteen million copies. Most self-made millionaires cite the book as being the foundation of their success.

Dr. Maxwell Maltz

A plastic surgeon in New York, Maltz was used to his patients' post-surgery reactions. In nearly all cases their self-esteem soared, yet for a small number, even though the cause of their low self-esteem had been removed, they felt no better.

This led to a long study of human nature and performance, building on the theories of 'self-consistency' by a Psychologist named Prescott Lecky.

Maltz's 1960 book, *"Psycho-Cybernetics"*[93], teaches the concepts of:

- self-affirmation,
- visualization,
- inner and outer goal-setting.

Not only has it helped millions of people in business and sport (notably the USA Olympic Teams), its theories underpin the work of most of the top motivation speakers, Zig Ziglar, Anthony Robbins, and Brian Tracy. Over thirty million copies have been sold.

The principles expanded in the three books are the core of every self-help book on the market and, although some of the 1930s & 1950s rhetoric should be taken with amusement, the core values are sound. There is no need to join a religion or cult to obtain these principles; if you are too lazy to read them you can find them as audiobooks.

The benefits of positive thinking translate into the way you do your job and your self-image. Your fellow crew members will be grateful of an enthusiastic colleague, one who is able to make the long night flights zoom-by.

This all helps you hit the pillow at night feeling good, and hence, able to achieve a better night's sleep.

Coffee

The stimulating benefits of caffeine are well-known for all night-flying air crew. There have been scientific studies documenting the effects of caffeine on the human body, its addictiveness (yes, try going cold-turkey and note the headaches, fatigue and muscle-pain), its nutritional value (zero), and its value as a stimulant (yes, but it doesn't replace sleep).

What you need to know, in relation to work, is this:

- It takes about fifteen minutes to half an hour to work,
- The half-life is six hours. That is, after six hours half is still in your system,
- If you are trying to use it to stay awake during a night flight, use it early. Do not wait until the head-nodding stage. From experience on the same flight leg, go for the coffee at a geographical location or time before you think you need a pick-me-up.
- Coffee is a diuretic. Which means it is useless in helping your body remain hydrated. You must drink more water than normal.

Bananas

For instant energy, useful before landing an aircraft in an emergency situation or to aid in having a clear head for the approach after a long night flight, have a banana.

Have two.

They are NOT diet food. *(Have you ever seen a skinny gorilla?)* One large banana contains 120 calories. That's about 20 more than Australia's favorite biscuit, the Tim Tam, (or two Oreo cookies for our American readers). And it has more fat and carbs as well.

But they work.

Amusingly, they also promote sleepiness. Have one after the coffee kicks-in.

Which Leg?

If you want to sleep within two hours of landing, choose the other leg.

Traditionally pilots fly leg-for-leg. That is, upon meeting at the briefing office the captain will ask the first officer which leg they would like fly. This supposes that there are no limits on weather or geography which require that the captain does a particular approach.

Helping make this decision are the familiarity with the route and destination, the weather involved or the difficulty of the radio procedures. The non-flying pilot handles all the radio communications so it may be prudent to get the pilot who is more experienced with the languages in question to do the radio work.

If you are planning on sleeping immediately after the last leg, then it may be prudent to fly the outbound of two legs. The brain activity required in handling the aircraft during the approach and landing is high and, for most pilots, it takes at least two hours to sleep afterwards. Better to let the other pilot do it if you plan on sleeping immediately after the flight, and handle the radio inbound instead.

RECAPPING:

- Developing an enthusiastic mental attitude helps yourself and your crew mates get through long boring flights. And a long career.

- There are a number of classic books (audiobooks) which help you get on well with other people:

    - *"Think and Grow Rich"*
        by Napoleon Hill

    - *"How to Win Friends and Influence People"*
        by Dale Carnegie

    - *"The New Psycho-Cybernetics"*
        by Dr.Maxwell Maltz

    - *"See You at the Top"*
        by Zig Ziglar

- It is possible to develop a healthy mental attitude without joining a cult.

- Strategically-used, coffee can help on long night flights. It's a diuretic though, so you need to drink more water.

- Bananas are an instant energy injection. Used with coffee, they can combat fatigue and increase performance.

- If you want to sleep within two hours of landing, fly the outbound leg.

From the Logbook

"A woman was attracted to a successful, highly-motivated, man. So much so that she invited him to visit during the afternoon when her husband was at work. They were in bed when suddenly she heard her husband's car in the driveway, she yelled:

'Quick! My husband is coming home!'

Her lover started putting on his clothes and said:

'Where's the back door?'

She looked startled and cried:

'We don't have a back door!'

To which the lover replied;

'Where do you WANT the back door?' "

So goes one of Zig Ziglar's yarns. If you ever have a chance to hear a recording of him giving one of his motivation lectures, take it. The 1974 book *"See You at the Top*[94]*"* (targeted at sales professionals and people who deal with others) has sold 1.4 million copies and countless audio tapes.

"The New Psycho-Cybernetics," an upgrade of the original work by Dr. Maltz, includes case histories and modern examples. After a business communication class my lecturer slyly opened his brief case and showed me his copy of *Psycho-Cybernetics*. Like a drug dealer he quietly said:

'You should get this ...'

Fearing that he was trying to get me to join the Scientologists I took off.

Only years later did I learn the difference between Maltz's *Psycho-Cybernetics* and the science fiction writer L. Ron Hubbard's foray into *'religion'* with *'Dianetics: The Evolution of a Science'*.

Crew Rest

Each airline and fleet has their own distinctive crew rest compartments. They can be in the roof as in the Boeing 777/787 and Airbus A350, rear roof and tail area as with the old Boeing 747, in the cargo compartments like the Airbus 340/A380, or in a huge box on a passenger deck as with another airline's A380. It's secret business, the crew rest compartment. No-one is allowed in there unless you are an operating crew or one of the cleaners. As with everything there is a procedure which must be followed.

Before flight the compartments are given the once-over by the crew. Emergency equipment checked, intercom handsets tested and a check to make sure that cleaners have installed the correct number of pillows and blankets. Hot-bedding is to be expected, but each crew gets to have their own pillow case and blanket. The augmenting flight crew-member carries out this role and makes their bed preflight. Often they will be going to bed as soon as the aircraft is above 10,000 feet, when the aircraft deck angle is still acute, therefore it's easier to perform this task on the ground.

The trick to surviving hours in crew rest is to not need to go to the toilet. If you are first into the bunk, slacken off your fluid intake in the hours before work. No tea or coffee. After your rest take as much water as you can. If you are second into the bunk, try to go easy on tea, coffee and water for the first half of the flight. The idea of crew rest is to sleep. It takes a few flights to get used to the claustrophobia (the beds are like coffins) and location. Jammed in the bulk cargo compartment, with the thousand kilometer per hour wind (620 mph) rushing past your head, your mind plays tricks. Dreams of fires, smoke, and gruesome crashes often haunt the newcomer. It gets better with experience.

In all airlines they have a tiny TV screen and a headset so you can watch a movie. Sadly, the person who put the screen in place had never tried to watch one while laid flat, thus failing to understand that the watcher needs to breathe more than once every movie. The reason you are there is to sleep and if sleep is not forthcoming, then you need to rest your eyes if nothing else.

For that reason, audiobooks are ideal and sometimes the droning voice may even put you to sleep.

Take the following into the crew rest compartment:

- A chocolate bar or banana. Something to eat when you wake-up.

- A small bottle of water.

- An iPod loaded with Absolute Sleep Music or equivalent, audiobooks, and earbuds.

- Earplugs and a sleep mask if they are not provided by the company.

- A silk sleeping bag liner, also called a travel liner. Some companies issue these along with crew pajamas, otherwise you can get one from an outdoor sports store.

Know the emergency equipment locations and procedures for getting out in a hurry.

Change into your company-supplied pajamas.

Use your blanket to cover the mattress. With your pajamas and the silk sleeping bag the chances are that the crew rest will get warm. Spend time getting your alarm clock right. Often it is easier to set a countdown timer.

Protocols allow that the flight deck may call you to wake you, or will send a crew member to wake you up. This involves a hand reaching in behind your curtain and give your leg a shake. *Here's hoping you will not be dreaming about a shark attack at the time.*

It is worth giving sleep a try, only reverting to audiobooks and finally, a movie, if sleep has eluded you.

Leave the crew rest area as you found it, preparing the area for the next crew, and being doubly sure to remove all food or drinks. Normally these are banned from the crew compartments. There are other crew in there, be respectful of their privacy.

RECAPPING:

- Know the emergency equipment and procedures for your crew rest.

- If you are first in, prepare your bed before take-off.

- Limit your liquid intake before your rest period to save having to get up and go to the bathroom.

- You will need:

    o Something to eat when you wake up halfway through your rest period.

    o A small bottle of water.

    o An iPod loaded with Absolute Sleep Music or equivalent, audiobooks, and earbuds.

    o Earplugs and a sleep mask if they are not provided by the company.

    o A silk sleeping bag liner.

- Take time setting your alarms or countdown timer.

- First, try to sleep. Resorting to audiobooks, music and finally, a movie only if sleep is not forthcoming.

From the Logbook

"William" was a First Officer who was flying on the 747. One day he was taking his rest and was summoned to the flight deck. A cabin crew was tasked with going into crew rest and waking the pilot.

Rather than calling out or knocking on the wall of his rest compartment, or reaching in and grabbing a foot and a shaking it, the crew member flung open the curtain without warning. Just as William reached the ultimate trajectory of a self-pleasure session.

The cabin crew received some of the results of his efforts upon their person.

The outcry that followed resulted in the unfortunate "William" being charged with sexual harassment. Unfairly suffering work-related stress and bullying, he eventually left his company and moved overseas to live. It is rumored that he even gave up flying.

For a time, whenever one of his company's pilots made an embarrassing or unprofessional radio call eliciting a groan *'What a wanker!'* often another pilot would key the mike and ask:

'William is that you?'

In the great Australian tradition of naming airway waypoints, he has been immortalized as a waypoint and standard terminal arrival route south of Melbourne.

May his (real) name live on forever.

Flight Deck Controlled Rest

The dictionary term of "profession" used to relate to lawyers, doctors, and theologians: people who had studied for years and made their income as standalone practitioners. *(Those in "The Oldest Profession" are another thing altogether ...)* Since pilots could never operate as their own business, only as wage-slaves to the airlines, they could hardly be seen as professionals.

They didn't have a university degree for a start, only a bunch of trade subjects. The last thing airlines wanted was a "thinking pilot" so instead employed glorified process-workers who, the aircraft manufacturers promised, could handle anything thrown at them. Even today, the main skill that pilots are selected for is "pattern-matching." They can quickly tell you what doesn't look right, memorizing complex processes and replicating them when requested. It's hardly *rocket-surgery.*

Universities have realized the cash-cow that is the Airline Transport Pilot License, and are wrapping up pilot training into "aviation degrees." But it's not a profession when compared to a lengthy medical degree followed by years to achieve specialization. Or the five years, including internship, to become a lawyer. Give the right person $120,000 and you can be an airline pilot in twelve to eighteen months.

Cabin crew are taken from customer service jobs and turned into security, safety and customer service specialists in less than two months. It's amusing to hear aircrew talking about "their profession" while exhibiting little in the way of a professional outlook.

They do not sleep before night flights, yet expect their colleagues to be well-rested, and even believe that they have a right to demand controlled-rest on the flight deck. Yet the laws in every regulatory state say something like:

"The pilot must be adequately-rested at the start of each duty period. During flights they must free from fatigue so as to operate at an optimum level of safety"

This law is then modified to appear in the company operations manual, each page of which is signed-off as an "Order," or amendment to the law, by the regulator. Every employee is required to obey the operations manual as it carries the full force of the law. Lawyers now make the employee sign-on electronically before each duty, ticking a box to agree with some vague statement that says they will operate to the conditions of the Operations Manual.

After the crash, if fatigue is a factor, the company has a ready-made statement:

'The pilot assured us he was fit and well-rested. If he lied, sue him.'

It can be cheaper for the company if the pilots can be found to have been at fault. These days, with massive improvements in air traffic systems, aircraft engineering and reliability, most crashes are pilot-caused.

Lawyers can make lots of money if they can convince the families of dead passengers to embark on huge class actions blaming the only two parties with money: the airline and aircraft manufacturer. The agony is prolonged for years in the hope that a single "magic bullet" will be found amongst the paperwork that proves the crash was caused by a mistake at the factory or airline.

Meanwhile, the company's New York lawyers are coming after you, the aircrew. In some jurisdictions you will be trying to prepare your case from behind prison walls since they lock-up witnesses first and ask questions later.

One legendary incident saw an airliner crash into terrain. The company's navigation department was at fault, but there was an effort to blame the pilots because a successful damages claim from the families of the more than two hundred and fifty victims would have bankrupted the airline. The airline was owned by the government of the small country, and a large payout per passenger would have done lasting damage to the treasury.

Even after an inquiry whose verdict was appealed to the country's highest courts, (in which the Royal Commissioner said he had been told 'an orchestrated litany of lies' by the airline), it came down to a court in New York to determine the cause of the crash that had occurred a decade earlier.

In amongst the duties of the New York court the case was slipped-in for judgement. Why? Jurisdiction, they successfully claimed. Was it that the aircraft manufacturer was from the U.S? Or because the aircraft was being handled by U.S. air traffic controllers when it crashed (even though they had been excused from giving evidence at all inquiries)? Or was it because of their insurers? Whatever.

The judge was bombarded with quotes from the previous inquiries, in which the chief pilot blamed the captain, then ruled it was caused by pilot error.

The verdict, among other things, included words to the effect:

'Because, as the Chief Pilot said, he was the Captain of the airliner and he should have known where he was at all times'

Kerching! Got 'em at last! Seat liability capped at around $40,000 per passenger and the airline survives to this day. They have, however, built an impressive shrine to the passengers and crew; and twenty years after the crash the airline's CEO apologized to everyone who did not receive appropriate support and compassion from the company following the crash.

Know that all your actions are going to be the focus of attention by some extremely erudite legal minds. You have a second to make a decision, perform an action and live with it. They will examine that decision, what led up to it, and its consequences for as long as they can. They are being paid by the minute and all of them have an addiction to German cars and children attending expensive schools.

This leads us to the issue. If you want to be treated as a professional, arrive at your airline well-rested and fit to do the maximum duty period, even if it is a quick out-and-back to a close port, because they can change your aircraft or flight destination and send you on a maximum duty flight. Weather and circumstances can further delay that duty, and they even have a nifty legal clause that allows them to extend your duty by a magical amount in order to complete the mission. Your two hour duty can turn into sixteen hours and include the most stressful event in your life. Are you ready?

Armed with that knowledge, you have arrived on the flight deck and for some reason you can't stay awake. Despite that the first page of your aircraft's flight manual introduces it as a "modern regular public transport two-crew airliner." Plus the fact that the passengers have paid serious money to obtain a ticket in an airplane with two pilots up front.

What do you think the passengers would say if you went down the back and asked them if they objected to your sleeping at the controls? Better still, imagine putting your most treasured family member on a flight, do you mind if 50% of the operating pilots on that plane were sleeping at the controls?

But you are going to have "controlled rest," even while knowing that all the other pilots (captains if you are a first officer and first officers if you are a captain) are raising you as topic of conversation at every barbecue. Why? *Because it is inconsiderate for the other pilot.*

While you are asleep they:
- Have to do your job,
- Cannot go to the bathroom,
- Have to wear a headset, and
- Cannot chat with the cabin crew (the cabin crew vanish when one pilot is asleep as they don't want to disturb him or her).
- Cabin crew are loathe to use the flight deck as relaxation to get away from the passengers for a break if they know one pilot is sleeping.

Since two thoughtful Northwest pilots overflew their home base while playing on their computers, we are no longer allowed to use our laptops or iPads to keep us alert. Now the FAA has banned us from taking photos from the flight deck.

The seconds drag around the dial and the flight drags on for everyone else. While you snore. Ever vigilant, your co-worker is waiting for the second when you have a nightmare and start kicking the rudder pedals. Those hot spots on your neck are the laser beam eye stares of your captain who, as a first officer would never have had the gall to suggest controlled rest "in the old days."

Do this:

- Do not take in-flight "controlled rest" unless you really need it.
- Be apologetic, recognizing that it is difficult for your co-workers.
- Give your colleague lots of time to prepare. They may wish to go to the bathroom or stretch their legs in the galley for a time. This may coincide with the crossing of a flight information region boundary or with obtaining an oceanic clearance. You will have to wait for that waypoint and then allow them to go out.
- Prepare for your return. Most companies allow a maximum of forty-five minutes "controlled rest" and you only want no more than twenty-six minutes for the Nasa Nap itself. Add a time marker or fix-info line into the flight plan's navigation display so that the other pilot knows when to wake you.
- Set an alarm in case your colleague falls asleep too.
- Write a sign "SPKRS OFF" and leave it on the pedestal as long as your speakers are turned down.
- Make sure that your rest period does not

coincide with:

- o the crossing of a flight information region boundary, or
- o area of severe weather, or
- o high minimum safe altitude airway, or
- o waypoint necessitating the obtaining of an oceanic clearance, or
- o a planned climb or descent point.

These areas are traversed quickly and it shouldn't delay your rest for long. Your consideration for the other pilot's workload will be mentioned glowingly at the next barbecue.

Some cabin crew baulk at bringing blankets and pillows into the flight deck as it concerns the first class passengers. Respect their position. Pilots often put their seat way back, and use their shoulder straps to restrain their crossed arms over their chests when sleeping. Earplugs and sleep mask are essential. A lumbar roll placed behind the neck can work wonders.

Recognize that, upon waking, your brain is mush for a few minutes. Factor that recovery time into the total rest period of about forty minutes. If you are still tired, recover for twenty minutes or so, then have another nap. The trick is to not enter REM sleep, lest the sleep hangover be worse than the cure. Etiquette dictates that when you have woken, restored your speaker position, and been briefed on the status of the flight; suggest that your colleague visit the restroom first.

What if it's not only you?

If it is a particular trip, or pairing of flights, or roster sequence that is causing pilots to require "in-seat relief," then it is important to file a Fatigue Report. The airline has been getting away with one fresh pilot covering for the other. But what happens if two hard-worked pilots are called from reserve to do the flight? What if both can't stay awake?

We know the answer to that.

After flying over just about every country ending in -*stan* without responding to radio calls, an Asian airline's 777 traversed the Black Sea and entered Bulgarian airspace. The two pilots woke with a start to see a MiG fighter on each side only meters from the cockpit window. Post 9/11, do you think authorities would allow a silent 777 to aim at a major city if there was no response from the crew, by interception signals, VHF, HF, acars, sat phone, or transponder?

If the pairing itself is the problem, go through the fatigue monitoring process. If a roster or pairing is 'dangerous' for you, it is for others as well. The only way to get it changed is by data accumulated by fatigue reports. Remember, we are dealing with accountants here. One airline with thousands of pilots is lucky to get six fatigue reports in six months, despite all the talk in the crew room and on the line by disgruntled pilots. When it comes to fatigue, it's a case of put-up or shut-up.

RECAPPING:
- **Ask yourself if you think it is professional to arrive for duty fatigued. If you are tired, stand your ground and go sick.**
- **Accept the consequences.**
- **Go through the fatigue monitoring process. If a roster or pairing is 'dangerous' for you, it is for others as well.**

- If, for some reason, you cannot stay awake, then Controlled Rest is a safer option.
- Be apologetic.
- Give your colleague lots of time to prepare.
- Make sure that your rest period does not coincide with:
  - the crossing of a flight information region boundary, or
  - area of severe weather, or
  - high minimum safe altitude (MSA) airway, or
  - waypoint necessitating the obtaining of an oceanic clearance, or
  - a planned climb or descent point.
- Add a time marker or fix-info line into the flight plan's navigation display so the other pilot knows when to wake you.
- Set an alarm, in case your colleague falls asleep too.
- Write a sign "SPKRS OFF" and leave it on the pedestal as long as your speakers are turned down.
- Move your seat way back. Use earplugs, eyeshades, a lumbar roll and maybe shoulder straps to help you sleep.
- Prepare for your return. Most companies allow a maximum of forty-five minutes "controlled rest" and no more than twenty-six minutes for the NASA Nap itself.

From the Logbook

Having been through an incident, an in-flight shutdown and diversion, the company safety department asked both pilots if they would mind their "running the process" for practice as, thankfully, they don't often get the chance. The pilots agreed and watched with interest as the investigator prepared the data from the quick access recorder. Software quickly merged the data and displayed it on an electronic google map. Impressive stuff. Every switch and lever position sampled, in some cases, every three seconds.

The interview. Question one:

'OK, before we start on the flight, let's go back two days before the flight. I wanna get a handle on what you ate and how you slept ...'

The correct answer, methinks, is NOT:

'Well, I was at a nightclub until 5 a.m. the day before the flight. Anyway, it's not my fault; I was asleep when the incident occurred ...'

Takeaway Ray was a colorful kleptomaniac, not a bad pilot though, and doing post graduate psychological research studies in his spare time. His career-ending thievery was rumored to include a small can of Diet Coke and a few packets of nuts.

Controlled Rest as a principle, came out the same month as a Notice To Pilots that we were no longer allowed to read newspapers on the flight deck.

He wryly observed:

'I'd much rather have to tell my F.O. *"Put down the newspaper, we're having an emergency!"* than have to wake him up.'

The NASA Nap

History's known nappers include Napoleon Bonaparte, Stonewall Jackson, Thomas Edison, Winston Churchill and Salvador Dali. U.S. Presidents John Kennedy, Lyndon Johnson and Ronald Reagan may all have achieved their success from having a daily nap. As has everyone who has had to fly an aircraft long haul, about two hours before sunrise. Should a pilot whose head was banging on their chest have a nap? What about Air Traffic Controllers?

The NASA Nap became known after a research project between NASA and some long haul airlines, one of whom was Air New Zealand. Seven hundred and fifty pilots were tested. During the study, in the early nineties, reports leaked stating that the most effective nap was one conducted "laid flat." That is, rather than sit at the control seat, pilots would be better to lie on the floor of the flight deck. However, today no written mention of this can be found. The results were released in 1995 which found that the ideal restorative nap was twenty-six minutes long. Subjects improved performance by 24% and alertness by 54%[95]. Any longer than twenty-six minutes and you chanced slipping over into the deeper REM sleep from which, if roused, you would suffer a sleep "hangover." A one hour sleep was in this category.

Studies found that people waking from a ninety minute sleep, the length of one sleep cycle, felt better than those roused from a sixty minute nap.

In a Stanford University study[96] forty-nine doctors and nurses were tested over three nights against a control group. About eight hours into their twelve hour shifts they were given a forty minute break, in which 90% received an average of twenty four minutes' sleep. Immediately after they woke they suffered short-term memory loss, but their overall performance was improved compared to the control group. At the end of their shift they undertook a forty minute "drive home" simulation. Their performance was no better than the control group.

MedicalDaily.com reported that Cambridge University studied daytime napping[97] and found that people who had a nap of longer than an hour a day had a higher than average risk of cancer, respiratory illness or heart attack. Over thirteen years they followed 16,000 people and while they reported on their napping and illnesses, they did not find a correlation between the two.

None of the studies delves deeply into the lifestyle variables in the subjects' lives before their duty period. Were they patients in retirement homes? What were their diets like? Were they smokers? Were they overweight? Did they undertake exercise? Did they get six to seven hours unbroken sleep in a dark, quiet room before their flight or emergency room duty? Were they suffering stress from family and other issues at the time? Were they taking medication? Did they receive healthy sun-exposure? What were their rosters like?

Thirty years in the industry cautions me into being skeptical.

The one thing that keeps recurring is that a nap *can* improve performance and alertness in the *short* term. How it effects your ability to land the aircraft in three hours has never been tested. A twenty-four to twenty-six minute nap should be followed by a non-duty period of about ten to fifteen minutes while the subject wakes up completely. This has been adopted by most regulators now as the industry standard for pilots as controlled rest. But not for air traffic controllers.

Despite three recent incidents in which American air traffic controllers fell asleep at their posts, their masters have rejected controlled rest techniques. Instead, they have employed more supervisors to watch the nodding heads.

RECAPPING:

- **A twenty-four to twenty-six minute nap improves performance and alertness.**

- **Most airlines adopting "Flight Deck Rest" expect that crew should have ten to fifteen minutes to properly wake up before resuming duties.**

- **There is no proof that a mid-flight nap helps with the landing or the drive home.**

- **If you are falling asleep while driving home, stop and have another nap.**

From the Logbook

To "spark-up" before going out to dinner, have a cup of coffee immediately before a twenty-five minute nap.

Set multiple alarms. Test to determine how long it takes your body to react to caffeine. You may discover that the nap and coffee helps more than either the nap or coffee alone.

The new Napwell Mask[98] may take napping to a new level.

At The Destination

Layovers can be the best part of the job, or the worst. Your choice.

Some crew seem to attack each destination like a travel writer on steroids, their lives a continuous blur of timetables and brochures; timed-to-the-second adventures where the actual flight is a slight inconvenience. Others become overwhelmed by exhaustion, don't prepare for the weather, forget to bring adequate clothing, and live on a diet of two minute noodles. At pickup they announce that they slept for twelve hours straight then couldn't get any sleep before the return flight.

A percentage remain in their room using the opportunity to study for their online university course, watch movies or read novels. Others have set routines for each destination, sleeping a couple of hours, then visiting the same restaurant, shopping for items to that city, or taking advantage of favorable exchange rates. For some the destination is home and their time is devoted to family and friends. You do not want to look back on your time in this industry and say to your grand-children that you never explored the famous cities of the world. Paris is one such destination. We stay at the airport and getting into the city is always a drama. In Paris, someone is always on strike. Most crew just stay in their rooms.

Have a plan of action. Spend money on taxis and go. It's much cheaper than coming back on holidays. You're staying in a five star hotel. Bite the bullet. Pay for a cab. When other crew members realize they can jump in the cab and share the fare, you will fill it up. Use your aircrew status and deploy some acting. Walk up to the box office of a show that's about to start, tell them you have just arrived in town, that you are a struggling air crew and ask if the producers have returned any *house seats* (used by the understudies and special guests). Wave cash, half the ticket price, and try your luck. You may find yourself six rows from the front, dead center and having a ball, sitting next to the next big name on Broadway.

Be careful of time zones. Falling asleep and dribbling on the shoulder of your neighbor is not classy. If you disgrace yourself apologize and say that you are a jet-lagged aircrew *from your opposition airline.*

Crew are given a cash allowance to cover the cost of meals. The airline expects you to eat in the hotel where the quality of the food is assured. Naturally crew like to pocket the money, instead surviving on two minute noodles or cheap street food. Reconsider, unless you are a local and know what to look for. As for noodles in polystyrene cups, the salt and MSG levels are high. There is about 80% of the daily sodium allowance in each cup, and they are high in mono sodium glutamate (MSG) which, although not going to kill you, can produce sleep-depriving side effects in some people.

You can sleep better on layovers if you:

- Never turn on the television (in case that horrible Sky News music is playing).

- Prepare for your departure as soon as you arrive. Hang up your uniform, get your next shirt ready, make it so you can wake up late and be racing out the door in seconds, worst case scenario.

- Order carbs. Your body will thank you for spaghetti Bolognese, something with rice or mashed potato. Layovers are all about comfort food that makes you sleep.

Bathroom

The layover starts as soon as the last passengers are off the inbound flight and you have completed the post-landing duties. Expect that there will be a long delay either in the airport or during your bus ride to the hotel and use the aircraft toilet. Even if you are staying at a nearby hotel your bus can breakdown and leave you stranded for an hour or so.

Cabin Bags

Keep close watch on your cabin bag. The best way for a spy to get things into a country would be to find a cabin crew bag near their seat, see which crew member owns it and then put the item in the bag. Chances are that crew member working in their section has their name emblazoned on their chest. Crew bags are rarely screened upon entry into a country and the bad guys know that.

It doesn't take much research to find out which hotel the airline uses. Then it's a matter of being in the lobby and watching the crew arrive and following the bag to a room. Even cleverer is to take a photo of the cabin crew during the flight and note their name. Upon arrival, SMS the picture and information to an accomplice who waits at the hotel check-in.

Following the cabin crew to their floor, as they are opening the door to their room, call their name to disarm them. Chances are they will be jet-lagged and expecting that, because you know their name, you are another crew member also staying at the hotel. The rest is easy.

So, if a customs officer asks:

'Has your bag been in your possession since it was packed?'

explain clearly that you packed it but *hundreds* of other people have had access to it. Then watch them call *Defor the Drug Dog* to have a sniff.

Going to your room

Assume that because you are in uniform and in the public gaze (some passengers photograph airline crew as they move *en masse* through the airport) you are being noticed. This may cause unwanted attention. While checking in don't loudly say your room number to other crew. Show your room number to your friend, they write it down, and you do the same with theirs. Go to the rooms in a group.

Some airlines have a policy of crew double-checking each other's rooms. That is, one crew stays in the hallway, the door is opened and a suitcase is jammed in the doorway. The other crew member enters and makes a security sweep of the room checking the bathroom, behind the drapes, and under the bed. Then the wardrobes. Check that the window is locked closed. Then the procedure is repeated for the crew member who stood guard.

Fires

No matter how tired you are it is important to do the next bit carefully. Most airlines have lost more crew in transport crashes and hotel fires than plane crashes. In a fire you can either survive or die, it's largely your call. Before you go into your room have a look up and down the hallway to see where your emergency exit is. Counting doors is a good idea, the next time you are out here the smoke may be ten centimeters (four inches) from the floor and it will be pitch black.

Saying out aloud to yourself the number of doors helps to imprint it into your brain:

'Turn left, across the hallway, 5th door.'

Look out the window. Could you jump in an emergency? First or second floor are an option. Third and fourth floor you can jump and survive but with broken bones. Above the fourth, no chance.

Transporting more people every day than airliners, trams, trains and buses combined, the humble elevator is the safest mode of transport. Each woven steel cable can support the car, and there are four or eight separate cables per car. They have two emergency braking systems in case all cables snap and a final buffer to ensure that a low altitude catastrophic failure's stop is smooth. But they can kill you in a fire.

The buttons, which work by the heat of a human finger, can be tricked by fire, calling the lift to the floor where the fire rages. Once the doors open smoke makes the sensors believe that someone is in the doorway and the doors refuse to close. Yet the chances of a lift catching fire are remote since, beside grease on the cables and pulleys, there is little to burn. Positive pressure fans may be used to ensure shafts are kept free of smoke, in the way they are used in stairwells. When the fire alarm is pressed, all the lifts return to the ground floor. When the firefighters arrive they are switched into manual mode and the firefighters use them to rescue people as well access the fire.

By the time you hear a fire alarm, you won't be using the elevator. The trip down the pressurized staircase may take half an hour, stopping every few steps as people join the exodus from floors below yours. It won't bother you, because you will already have planned what you are going to wear in case of an evacuation, won't you? Standing around in the street for three hours waiting for the all-clear is embarrassing in nothing but bare feet and underwear.

There is a great deal of information about surviving hotel fires and you should do your own research if it is not part of your airline's training course. Suffice to say that you can *sleep* better if you can fully relax. And you will, knowing that your fire safe procedures are in place.

Room Security

The *"Do Not Disturb"* sign goes on the door as you are walking in and the chain or secondary lock goes on in one movement. Bad guys know that this is the time that guests can easily be disorientated. If you hear a quick knock on the door:

'Excuse me, engineering, I left some tools in the room...'

immediately after you have closed the door and slid the chain, your brain will think something is weird. Yell out to hang on and ring the front desk to ask security to come up. A real engineer will understand and enjoy the break. If he makes a fuss, even more reason to *not* let him in.

Upon Entering

Put your room key in the same place in every room you visit. That way it will fall easily to hand if you have to leave in an emergency. Have a plastic loyalty card, or comb, that you can jam into the hotel's key holder to turn on the electricity to the room. This way the air-conditioning, lights, and television stay on if you go downstairs. Sometimes only the hotel's room card will work. In this case, leave it in position and get a new one from the front desk. Get the luggage rack and assemble it. Remember that bed bugs are your enemy. Keep your suitcase up off the floor, away from fabrics, and closed between 10 p.m. and 6 a.m. See that the room temperature can be controlled and set it now; it saves re-packing if you have to change rooms later.

Take the filthy bedspread (counterpane) off and wrap it up. Most hotels only wash them four or five times a year, and most guests put their suitcases, among other things, on them. Check for bed bugs. Lift up the bedding of the head end corner and closely inspect the mattress joins. If there are signs, you won't be staying here.

Think about security, both in the room and if you are planning on going out. Having a small wallet with a few notes and maybe a few loyalty cards in a back pocket might save your day. 'Here, take it!' Throw it in their face and run. Seeing the prize of credit cards and notes floating towards them distracts even the toughest thief. Meanwhile your front pocket contains bills, a credit card, the room key and piece of torn-off stationary with the hotel's name and address on which you have written your room number. It helps the emergency room nurses do their job, and you too, if you become disorientated.

In every new and strange city, expecting that you are being followed and targeted allows you to abruptly stop or change direction. Look at people long enough to study their description. The bad guys are looking for victims who are oblivious to security, who won't even know they have been robbed, let alone put up a fight. As soon as you act aware and differently you drop off their radar. There are plenty more fish in the sea for them.

Everything of value goes into the hotel safe. Make up an inventive pin number for the safe, bits of your staff number or start date; not the usual 12345. It's been done before.

Going Out

As you leave your room, talk as you open the door:
'OK, you can stay up for another thirty minutes ...'
or
' ... alright then, I'll back in a few minutes,'
clearly giving anyone loitering in the hall the impression that there is someone in the room. Leaving the television on also does the trick, with the risk that you will begin watching it upon your return. You will develop your own routine in time. Many people go to hotel gyms; others, who use the gym at home instead use the layover as a treat and obtain their exercise by walking.

One friend walks the Thames River during his London layovers. It has been a destination of his for over twenty years and there's not much of the city that he hasn't explored. Each trip he catches a train to where he finished walking last trip, and resumes his trek. After a few hours he either finds another train, or pub, or catches a cab back to the hotel.

Walk, run, jog, shuffle, skip, ride or stretch. Whatever your method, layovers are a time to get some exercise. Make sure you have good footwear. You don't want to get an injury, and you're less of a target if you can sprint away from trouble. Nothing attracts attention more in a big city than someone running flat-out, except someone running yelling "Fire" or, in America, "Gun."

If your flights take you west, a long morning walk during your home time zone means that you will be exploring the destination during the sunrise, known as the photographer's hour. Being in place to capture the first rays ensures great images, from Sydney Harbor, to the Great Wall, Hong Kong to New York. You hardly have to be an expert. Concentrate on having things in focus with the rising sun over your shoulder. The benefit from the exercise, followed by a carbohydrate-laden breakfast/lunch, is that you get to sleep four to six hours before the return flight. Provided, that is, you substituted hot chocolate or chamomile tea for coffee after your walk.

With everything ready to go and multiple alarms in place, never having to rely on the hotel wake-up call, you should be able to relax sufficiently to sleep. The ultimate goal is to wake up naturally after six hours sleep, about two minutes before the cacophony of alarms go off. If you plan your layovers, take the right clothing, adopt wise security measures, plan for disasters and develop simple strategies when it's only a mental exercise, get into wise habits and be assertive; you will find that you feel more in control.

And you'll *sleep* better, even in the city that never sleeps.

RECAPPING:

- Plan for your layover.
- Take the right clothing for the forecasted weather.
- Check out what shows and events will be on.
- Always visit the bathroom before you leave the aircraft.
- Keep an eye on your cabin bag/nav bag and tell Security or Customs that people may have tampered with it.
- When checking-in be aware that people are watching.
- Don't yell out your room number.
- Go to your room with another crew member if possible.
- Be suspicious of anyone in the hallway as you approach your room. If in doubt, keep walking.
- Do a quick room sweep.
- Locate your nearest fire escape and say it aloud to yourself.
- Place the Do Not Disturb sign on the door and set the safety catch as soon as you are inside and expect that *The Bad Man* will immediately knock on the door. Don't be fooled.
- Leave your room key in the same spot.
- Check that you can control the temperature.
- Perform a quick bed-bug search.
- If you are staying, erect your suitcase stand, away from curtains and fabrics.
- Make up a "robber's wallet" with some old loyalty cards and some low denomination bills.

- Check out the safe and put passport and other valuables inside.
- Only leave those items outside the safe that you are prepared to live without.
- Choose a proper PIN number for the safe. At least, make it a challenge for the thief.
- Leaving the room, exit quickly, while talking back to the room. Leave the TV on.
- In a foreign city, choose footwear in which you could sprint twenty meters if needed, and study possible pickpockets.
- Do the unexpected now and then, turn back to study a store window, change sides of the streets. Go into a shop.
- In places where the language is foreign, get someone on the front desk to write the address on hotel stationery so a taxi driver can bring you back.

From the Logbook

Jumping from above the fourth floor of a building is mostly suicide, unless your name is Sebastian Reyes[99], who after a night of partying in July 2015, fell off a balcony seventeen floors up. The energy of his fall was broken by a car shelter, the car parked underneath, its front suspension and the air in the front tires. His spectacular arrival was filmed by CCTV. He woke up in hospital with a broken thigh and pelvis. *They always say that God protects drunks.*

The winter bus rides in Moscow are legendary: three hours is not uncommon. In Seoul, I have been stuck in the bus for two hours forty-five minutes during torrential rains with flooding.

In New York, we once spent two hours getting from the airport to the hotel; while a friend told me the one hour bus ride in Manila turned into three hours and forty-five minutes with no possibility of a toilet stop for three hours.

We had been warned that a particular hotel's staff were stealing from crew who had left valuables in their rooms. Not from the room safes but from the rooms themselves, which begs the question: *"Why weren't valuables in the safe?"* In an effort to dissuade the thief I removed two pages of A4 from my bag.

On one I wrote:

SMILE!
You are LIVE
on RoomCam.com

It was left propped up on the upturned waste bin that I placed on the desk chair inside the door. Blue-tacked to the outside of the door, above the "Do Not Disturb" sign, the other sheet was emblazoned with:

LIVE ROOM CAM
VIDEO IN PROGRESS
DO NOT ENTER

I never got robbed.

Security is all about doing what everyone else isn't. It's much easier for a professional thief to target someone who has no idea. They will be carrying more cash and will not put up a fight. Their powers of observation are useless and they will be unable to give a description.

On a recent trip to placid Melbourne I returned from an afternoon out to see a lady being interviewed by four police in the foyer. As I went past I noticed that her statement had run a full page in the policewoman's notes.

I later found out that it was one of our crew who had arrived from a later flight, exhausted, and a man had tried to grab her as she was entering her room. She screamed, fought like a tiger and did the last thing he'd expect, dropped her suitcase and took off down the hallway.

He was never seen again.

One thing is for sure: *it would have taken her a long time to get to sleep after that experience.*

Jet Lag

In a discussion about jet lag we have to weed out the word *jet*. Talk descends into a discussion of how to have a more comfortable flight IN the jet which is an important, but separate, issue that we'll deal with in the bonus chapter *"23 Tips To Survive A Long Flight."* Jet lag has to do with the sun, the planet and your position on it. And how fast you get from one place to the other. It's a coincidence that the jet engine has made it possible to be a problem for people other than Russians.

Russians? Well, in history, no other country spans so many time zones. Trying to trick time they have moved from sixteen time zones to eleven 'real' zones. In an effort to make life easier they now have permanent daylight saving which is now their standard time.

Jet lag was a problem for the huge country, close to the Arctic Circle, in that you could buy a ticket on the Trans-Siberian Express from Moscow to Vladivostok and start heading east at 100 kph (62mph), then keep going for one hundred and forty three hours and twenty minutes. In every other country an ocean would have got in the way. You'd have to adjust to it being seven hours earlier when you got out of the train. Your body would still think it was midnight but the sun would be coming up which is made even creepier to the passengers because all railways in Russia run on Moscow time as it is easier to run the trains that way.

In the same way all pilots fly on one time zone: Greenwich Mean Time (which became Co-Ordinated Universal Time in 1961 then, to appease the French six years later: Universal Time Co-Ordinated), or UTC. It's only passengers and airports that run on local time. Which is why you sometimes hear pilots giving a public address, letting the passengers know that they are arriving more than an hour early or late. Then instilling a terrifying confidence by adding …

'Um, er, that can't be right…'
Leading half the passengers to wonder:
'Oh My God! If he can't even tell the time, how the hell is he gonna land the plane?'

Jet lag is a circadian rhythm problem for humans who are affected by the way the sun shines relative to their established body clock. It's a lesser issue for some blind people, notably the late Ray Charles who stressed-out promotors by refusing to arrive in the city until near the time of his concerts, citing:

'Blind people don't get jet lag. Why do you want me to sit in a hotel room for an extra day?'

Most blind people *are* affected by jet lag, but to a lesser degree than sighted people.

With lives also regulated by the sun, animals must also be affected by jet lag. There is some evidence that race horses can gallop for up to twenty-four seconds longer before fatigue sets in after a long flight. Whether that has to do with jet lag or the exhilaration of not being cooped-up in a plane can never be known.

We get jet lag by crossing time zones in jets. If teleportation, favored by science fiction writers, had taken off before jets then it'd be called 'teleport lag' if you quickly crossed time zones.

So what's a time zone? Imagine planet earth. Now put yourself at the top at the True North Pole, where the imaginary pole exists around the axis of rotation. You could stand right on the top. Every direction would be south and you could walk around in circles crossing every time zone in seconds. Well, you could if it was on land. But it's in the middle of the Arctic Ocean where the sea is 4,261 meters (13,980 feet) deep. The nearest land, an island off Greenland, is about 700 kilometers (435 miles) away. Sure, there's shifting pack ice but it's easier to perform this trick at the South Pole where the Americans have a base and every direction you look, with your back to the pole, is north.

After "running around the world" you could go inside for a cup of hot chocolate, a clever idea considering the winter low is -60 Celsius (about -76 Fahrenheit) for six months of the year. Compared to only -57 Celsius (-71 Fahrenheit) where airliners cruise.

Grab an orange. For argument's sake it is now planet earth. Looking down on it you would be confronted with a basic circle, widest at its 'equator.' You could draw a line around the equator. Circles are distinctive because they are divided up into 360 degrees. If we wanted we could put 360 evenly-spaced marks around the equator. We know that the earth rotates completely every twenty-four hours, counter-clockwise if you are looking down on it. 360 degrees divided by twenty-four hours equals fifteen degrees. Therefore, at the equator, if you went east for fifteen degrees and stopped, you would notice that the sun rose and set an hour earlier, and so on, all the way around.

For fun, on your orange, you could count off these fifteen degree marks and draw a line from one pole to the other, crossing the marks. In the end you would have twenty four segments, fattest at the equator and each converging to a point at each pole.

[Right now, for research purposes, you are considering getting a Terry's Chocolate Orange ball to prove it. I just did. But instead of 24 there are only 20 segments ... no, make that nineteen. *OK, eighteen ... What? Only six left?*]

Each one of the LONG lines is called a line of LONGitude. And each one is, for time zone purposes, one hour ahead of (or behind) the one beside it. You can appreciate that running up and down one of the lines will not change your time, relative to when the sun comes up. That's going from the top (north) to the bottom (south) and as long as you stay on your segment, your time doesn't change.

Even if you fly for fourteen hours from Moscow to Johannesburg, despite changing from summer to winter or vice versa, your time, relative to sunrise, doesn't change. No jet lag. You still are going to feel like you have been run over by a truck, but that is for the bonus chapter. It is only when you go from east to west (sideways) that you start crossing the time zones, start playing tricks on your body and affecting your sleep.

How long it takes to cross those time zones depends on your LATITUDE. For some obscure reason I remember latitude as FATitude because the planet is fatter than it is high, by 42.72 kilometers (26.54 miles). At the equator, the earth is rotating at 1,674 kph (1,040 mph). At Kennedy Space Centre, 31% of the way to the North Pole, it's still doing 1,470 kph (913 mph) which is a significant free ride when you're shooting rockets to fly around the planet.

The further you go towards the poles, the slower the rotation. At the South Pole you could go and stand a hundred meters away and it would take twenty-four hours to get back to the same spot. *[Forgetting the fact that earth would be 2,592,000 km (1,610,591 miles) further along its annual trip around the sun.]*

Eighty degrees north or south of the equator (ten degrees from the poles) is still too cold for humans, being only 1,111 km (690 miles) away, but at this distance the earth's rotational speed is noticeable at about 290 kph (180 mph). About sixty degrees north, where we find Québec, St. Petersburg and Scotland's Shetland Islands you are heading eastward at a lazy 835kph (518 mph) which makes for relaxing sunrises and sunsets, unlike the "lights on, lights off" shock that greets first timers holidaying near the equator. *You have to be quick if you want to share a romantic sunset in Singapore.*

The width of a time zone segment at the equator is 1670 km (1037 miles), and half that at St. Petersburg. Another reason why it's easy to cross so many zones in Russia. At those latitudes the distances are manageable. The more time zones you cross, the more your body is going to be confused when you stop. And while you can get used to the changes through education and experience, you can't stop getting jet lag. It is a badge of honor, proving that you have indeed, circumnavigated the planet. It's only proper that you feel different. Millions before you died trying to do what you just did.

The effects are worse heading east, as you "lose" time. Seven hours' time difference from the Middle East to Australia's east coast and you are ready for bed when everyone, the sun included, is getting up. Your body feels cheated and misses out on sleep. Heading west, say from the Middle East to New York, your day goes on forever. You 'make' time. After twelve hours of travelling it's still mid-afternoon. You hit the hotel room and, as the sun goes down, you happily fall asleep.

The effects of jet lag vary, but they break down into three groups:

- Physiological
- Mental
- Sleep

Physiological

Your body behaves as it would in the old time zone when you are in another. It takes a day to catch up one or two time zones. A London to Sydney trip will take about five to six days to adjust. As well as constipation and/or diarrhea, first timers at long haul travel never fail to notice that their bowel movements now occur at different times of the day. For someone who has always had a morning bowel movement, it can be disconcerting that this now occurs in mid-afternoon, or last thing at night.

One high-flying VVIP business mogul tries to beat this by having nothing in his bowel during a flight. He is so convinced that a clean bowel is the key to beating jet lag that he has a colonic irrigation session prior to each long haul flight in his corporate jet. He is in his 80s, so who's to say it doesn't work?

The Mayo Clinic website provides healthy skepticism by suggesting that the human body, well nourished, is perfectly good at ridding itself of waste. And has been for centuries. A lubricated firehose, no matter how well-meaning, should not be introduced into the area.

Irritability, nausea, sweating, dehydration, and headaches are not caused by jet lag but by the mode of transport. As are the muscle cramps, and menstrual problems.

If you could transit the same number of time zones without the:

- Departure airport experience
- Stress of leaving
- Rapid temperature changes
- Claustrophobic experience
- Mild hypoxia
- Mild deep vein thrombosis
- Arrival airport experience,

then most symptoms attributed to jet lag would be eliminated. And can be for the seasoned traveler.

Mental

The mental fuzziness, confusion, and problems trying to concentrate on the simplest of tasks seem to be jet lag related. No matter how well you travel, chances are that you find yourself making silly mistakes upon arrival. With that in mind, do not hire a car at Los Angeles airport after a fifteen hour flight and plan to do battle with the peak hour traffic if you have never driven on the right hand side of the road before. Hire car companies report that most of their customer crashes occur within twenty minutes of the LAX car parks.

Be wary about signing important deals or contracts when you are expecting to be jet lagged. Go over the contract details before you leave instead and, if necessary, walk straight into a meeting from the plane. But be wary of the dreaded *third day.*

For large time zone changes the third day is when your body gives up trying to play the game. When you least expect it an overwhelming tiredness hits you. Give in and sleep as long as you need. Plan for it by clearing your diary in advance. Pushing through, using caffeine and will-power, is an option. Apologize to your family, friends and work colleagues in advance. You will be crabby. Sadly for aircrew, the third day often coincides with their next trip. Luckily for us, since we were only on the other time zone for a brief stay, our jet lag is not as pronounced as the relocating expat passenger or holiday-maker.

Quite often we will stay on our home time zone, which is quite acceptable with 24 hour room service. It astounds even the most seasoned aircrew when arriving in USA hotels that room service is usually closed from midnight to six in the morning. You do, however, always have access to an ice machine. *How do I know? My room is always next to it.*

Sleep

Often the first time a person experiences insomnia is when suffering from jet lag. Being dog-tired yet unable to sleep, rolling around in a hotel bed knowing that your arm has NEVER been in this position before in your whole life. (*"How did I ever sleep with THIS hanging off my neck?"*) Other times you crash so hard before you undress, or turn off the television or lights, waking with a cricked-neck, pounding headache, and that bloody Sky News theme. Or you're like a petulant three year old, snapping at family members, and then falling asleep at the dining table. Worse, you know that you are behaving like a shit, and can't help yourself.

On day three, don't make appointments or important plans. Be ready to give in, whatever time it hits you. If it's a mid-afternoon nap that lasts eight or ten hours, so be it.

Jet lag cures

Nothing can be taken to speed up the joining of your body with your new location on the planet except for time, water and sunshine. Take as much of each as you need. A cup of tea and a sit in the sun, with a cat or puppy on your lap, is all you need. The general rule is that you should stay up until local bedtime, which may be difficult if you have been flying all night and landed at dawn. In that case, grab a few hours' sleep and force yourself to wake after a few hours.

Get onto your new time zone, psychologically, as soon as you can. Up to a week ahead, start bringing your sleep earlier if you are headed east. Listen to destination radio stations on TuneIn Radio and be aware of their local time. Read their newspapers online and start following the local issues. Put your watch on destination time at the start of the flight.

Understand that no pills, or magical cures can hasten recovery. There is an entire industry trying to convince you otherwise. They are wrong, and are all trying to rip you off. Be kind to yourself and your wallet. If you are aircrew embarking on a long haul career, understand that while you can learn to manage it, or rather, *your personal reactions to shifting time zones,* you can't BEAT it.

So stop trying.

RECAPPING:

- Jet lag has to do with crossing the time zones, then stopping.

- It has physiological effects, your body's rhythms and cycles continue in the old time zone and take a day for each one or two time zones travelled, to catch up.

- It has mental effects, your brain is certain that it is midnight but the sun is coming up.

- Your brain can be extremely alert one second and fuzzy the next.

- Be extra careful of driving immediately after arrival. You have no spare capacity and are only surviving on experience. Especially if everyone else appears to be driving on the wrong side of the road.

- Expect that your arrival will result in sleep issues and be ready to react accordingly.

- The rule is that you should stay up until local bedtime, get exercise, water and sunshine.

- The dreaded Third Day can see you fall asleep in flash. Plan for it and give in. Sleep as long as you need.

From the Logbook

I come from the land down under, where we drive on the left side of the road. When I am in countries that drive on the left I only drive manual cars. When I am in right hand drive countries I only drive automatic cars, realizing that when I have an emergency behind the wheel I will not have the years of subconscious experience to help me. Knowing this, I limit the amount of brain capacity needed to drive.

Our first flights to New York saw us arriving about 2 p.m. local which, to us, was 11 p.m. No matter what we did, we were asleep on our feet by 9 p.m. local.

At 4 a.m. we were wide awake, when the only thing open was the diner behind the hotel, and the Apple store. Drinking their coffee at the diner, cops would sit watching the only life visible on the streets: a steady stream of wide-eyed aircrew coming back from the Apple store with the distinctive white shopping bags.

When we first started flying the large airplane from the Middle East the only destinations were the U.S.A., and Australia. For two years our body clocks were between Bali and Singapore or between Iceland and Greenland. Never in the same place as our bodies.

Hundreds of pilots and cabin crew missed birthdays, medical and dental appointments, dinner parties, lunch catchups and everything in between.

Were we sleeping?

Nope, just lying on the couch staring at Mega Machines, Air Crash Investigations, and MythBusters. Too trashed to change channels, even though the remotes were in our hands.

Jet lag is like that.

Jen and Jim are a retired Australian couple who were on last leg of their "world tour of churches" (or so it seemed to Jim). They arrived in America, where people drive on the wrong side of the road.

Severely jet lagged, and a nearing the limit of his politeness, Jim drove out of the rental car park immediately onto the majestic American highway system. For first timers it is awe-inspiring. Within seconds you forget about where you are meant to be going, swept along in a tsunami of cars.

Eventually spying his exit he made it onto the off-ramp that soon became one of those freeway cloverleaf affairs that Australians had only seen on Bugs Bunny Cartoons.

He and Jen weren't on speaking terms at that stage, when his hand brushed the steering wheel indicator stalk.

The previous hirer of the car must have been running late to get to the airport and previously set the cruise-control to warp speed. It now re-engaged.

Never having used cruise-control in his life, Jim had no idea why, entering a 270 degree turn, his car should decide to automatically accelerate to the speed-of-sound. Steering suddenly occupied all his attention.

As sweat instantly broke out from every pore, Jen was sitting, arms crossed in the passenger seat thinking:

'You can't scare me!'

About halfway around the turn he found the brake pedal, which disconnected the cruise control.

You can still drive a car with jet lag, but have little spare capacity for anything else.

… Amazingly, they are still married.

I am thinking of starting a kitten and puppy rental service for jet lagged aircrew. You get back from a trip, and dial 888, *Paws&Tea Jet lag Rescue*.

A vehicle resembling an ambulance speeds through the city and comes to your house. Doors open and two uniformed experts set you up with a comfortable deck chair in the sunshine. One puts a puppy in your lap while the other makes you a cup of tea.

Then they are off to respond to other calls.

After an hour or so they return to rescue the poor animal and replace it with a fresh one. They might even care enough to make you another cup of tea.

The Expatriate Lifestyle

Thousands of people in this industry have to relocate in order to gain or continue their employment. The time given to relocate and set up is limited as the companies are interested in having you online and being productive as soon as possible. It may only be a matter of weeks from your first interview and/or simulator check to relocation, medicals, ground school, and simulator training.

As well as the stress of leaving home, packing up, and a long flight, jet lag may kick in during the same time when you are making important decisions. It's worse if this is your first "expatriate" (expat) experience. Old hands who have had to set up house in new countries more than a few times are wise to the tricks. Sometimes it is easier in a country where most of the labor is expat and everyone you meet has been where you are now. In my Carrefour supermarket in the Middle East you can always see a dazed-looking person with a clothes airing rack jammed into their oversized trolley. You feel like saying:

'Welcome! The shower curtains are over here.'

We've all been there.

Firstly, don't panic. Do one thing at a time and ask for help, *'Where do I find ...?'* There's always a kind heart ready to help.

Secondly, establish clear priorities. One guy who was embarking on his first expat move was more preoccupied with getting a brand new vehicle, which required a bank account, driver's license and insurance. Meanwhile, he was failing to hit the marks in the first important week of ground school. He was getting noticeably stressed to the level that onlookers were concerned that he would find himself with a car, but no job.

Large airlines expect you to hit their marks:

- Pass the medical
- Pass the ground school.
- Pass the simulator program.
- Pass the line training.
- Pass the line check.

Exhaustion will eventually make you sleep like a baby. When you have secured the job, only then consider that you might be staying in your new land.

Finally, set yourself up. You can live inexpensively in the world but there are a few things on which you should splurge:

Excellent medical insurance

Depending on your location, a fly-out facility to a nearby first-world country may be prudent. If you are working on a contract, and don't trust your agency, consider this: even though they offer medical insurance, is it the type of insurance you need? And do you think that they will be able to pay the premiums every month?

For one contract I was dubious. The month you need to be flown out of a third world country could also be the month they forgot to pay the bills. I cocktailed-up my own insurance using a broker in my home country using TWO companies. If one went under, I was still covered. Expensive, but I slept better.

Top quality internet

The fastest that you can get. Optical fiber to the lounge room if possible. You can put up with changed rosters and annoying local difficulties if you can escape via the web.

Top cable television

Being able to keep in touch with your favorite programs and sports from home lessens the stress.

No expense-spared communication

To be able to speak to your family, or video conference, using Skype or FaceTime, anytime you want. A virtual private network (VPN) may be recommended in areas where internet security is not assured, especially for when doing internet banking. Witopia.com[100] has proven reliable over the last decade.

Turning the inside of your expat abode into a haven from home is one way of dealing with the difficulties of living in a land of different languages and customs, even religion. And nothing is more sacred than the bedroom. Spend money on a good bed, air-conditioning/temperature control, double-glazing, soundproofing if necessary, blackout blinds and at least one blackout curtain.

Establish a doable exercise regime to ensure regular sleep. Being sleep-deprived is not clever in a foreign country if, say, you are riding a motor scooter to work.

It's one thing to visit these places as a tourist, but as an expat everything changes. Getting a phone or internet connected can do your head in. Registering a car. Buying insurance. It all becomes harder when you don't speak the language. Journalists use "fixers" in each country they touchdown. These are people who are trusted with providing the right drivers and vehicles, who have done the pre-production, lined-up interviewees and so on.

In your destination you will soon find a fixer. Ask around. There will be an MBA student who wants to practice his or her English on you. Come up with an arrangement that if they can arrange something for you, cable TV for example, then you will pay them on performance. The cheaper they can negotiate it for you, the more you pay them. The faster it can be up and running, the more they get.

Soon you will be getting deals all over town that the other expats could only dream about, plus you will be moving within local circles and get to enjoy your time more than the expats who lock themselves away after work. Some of your most memorable times will be dining in the homes of the locals, being treated fondly by whole families (even if it is so they can laugh at you).

Back in your house, TuneIn Radio[101] on iPads and smartphones allows you to choose radio from all around the world. Keeping in touch with radio and news from home helps with homesickness and allows you to carry on knowledgeable conversations with friends and family back home.

PressReader.com[102] allows you to read newspapers from all over the world, as their editors intended, for the price of one newspaper subscription.

WhatsApp[103] allows you to send SMS, pictures and sound bites in a family ping pong game that is never ending.

Skype and FaceTime, used for long periods in conference mode, can make you feel like you are in the other room.

Facebook and Twitter can become full-time jobs, if you let them. Since you are *trying* to keep in touch, you find that you are in contact with your family and friends much more than if you had stayed at home.

At some stage treating yourself to an over-the-top present; a super TV, expensive boat or car; appears to be the right thing to do. Try to think carefully about it, asking yourself if you would even think of taking this course of action back home.

Pilots have motto,

'If it flies or floats ... hire it.'

If you do an analysis on the hours of pleasure versus the hours getting ready, cleaning, storing etc., you may find it easier to hire, then walk away. Expats buying "toys" as a present for their loneliness or "martyrdom" can lead to a decade or more overseas with nothing to show for it. It has been the reason of more than one expat divorce.

Be prepared to make adequate sleep your most important non-work activity. Instead of drinking to excess every night, happily leave parties early, waving:

'It's past my bedtime!'

as you take your leave. Let it become a standing joke. Being able to sleep when you want is the mark of a Professional Sleeper. Considering you are going to sleep for fifty years before the "Big Sleep" starts, it's not a bad thing to be good at.

RECAPPING:

- Don't panic. Few things have to be done at once.

- Ask for help. Enlist in the services of a local to help you.

- Prioritize. Secure the job first. Hit the marks at work.

- Obtain excellent medical insurance.

- Arrange top quality internet access.

- Get cable television.

- Spare no expense on communication, which may require joining Witopia and getting a Virtual Private Network.

- Spend money on making your bedroom sound and light proof.

- Use TuneIn Radio and PressReader to keep in touch with home.

- Make WhatsApp, Facebook and Twitter an important part of your life to keep in touch.

- Don't fall into the expat traps of buying expensive toys and developing a drinking habit.

- Make adequate sleep your goal.

From the Logbook

In 2004 after six months living in the suburbs of Ho Chi Minh City, Vietnam, I finally convinced the phone company to connect the internet to my place. This resulted in a team of guys in bright blue overalls and orange hard hats arriving in my street after they had strung the LAN cable all the way from the exchange. The cable was as blue as their uniforms.

The whole street came out watch. Eventually the end of the cable was brought to my modem and plugged-in. The workers were impressed when it worked.

Within the crowd of spectators were some wise souls who lay backwards on their motorcycles, smoking, as they looked up at the wires and contemplated the dilemma.

Could they hook into my LAN cable as successfully as they had done to my electricity?

The bonus chapter

23 Tips to Survive a Long Flight
(As a Passenger)

A wise old aviation medical examiner sat looking thoughtfully then raised his head. In his thick Welsh accent he proclaimed:

'The granny you put onto a plane in London is NOT the same little old lady who gets off the plane in Melbourne.'

Long haul flying wears you out, *regardless* of the direction and time zones crossed, if any. And then jet lag knocks you around afterwards. How can you get into a situation where the flight is less of a harrowing experience? And have a better quality of sleep before, during and after the flight?

1. The reason we fly

Having been in the game for thirty years it's sad to look back and see the *"de-aviation"* of the flying experience. Nowadays when we push-back into our own exhaust fumes, and that marvelous kerosene smell fills the cabin, we can guarantee a worried call from the cabin crew advising us of the fumes. When we were kids we used to go to airports to sniff the kerosene on the breeze. The Jet-A1 got into our blood and we became aviators.

Today the terminal is air-conditioned and the aerobridge/jetbridge is fireproofed, guaranteed to prevent the ingestion of flames or fumes from the tarmac. And now most people couldn't tell you what brand of aircraft they were in until they read the safety card. If they read it at all.

It's all about marketing, destinations, saving money, collecting points, watching movies and having a *"restaurant experience."* Why? Because the airlines don't want you to think about what, in fact, is really happening. Only meters away there is a blast furnace or two, white hot metal spinning within a few centimeters of a swimming pool full of volatile fuel. The takeoff roll sees you going faster than a formula one car, and then it starts to speed up. You're doing 500 kph (310 mph) in minutes.

In the cruise the air's so cold, only a few centimeters from your face, that you would snap freeze. You're going so fast that the wind would strip off your clothes, and, if you opened your mouth, your skin. The engine noise would deafen you.

There haven't been recent studies, but in 2007 the New York Times reported that the American National Institute of Mental Health had put the number of Americans who suffered 'aviophobia' at 6.5%[104]. Yet a broader study done in Australia during the early 1980s reflected that half the general public was *'too scared to fly.'* Whatever the real figure, the concept of flying is stressful for a percentage of people. The physics involved is beyond the understanding of nearly all the passengers and most of the people who work in the airline. Yet they roll up on the jetbridge, eager to get on.

Or do they?

On every flight there are terrified travelers, first-time fliers, people fleeing a horrible past, grandparents looking forward to seeing their grandchildren for the first time, uncertain people travelling to a new city for a new life, unaccompanied kids (the airborne balls in a game of Family Law ping-pong), sad lovers, happy lovers, expectant mothers, those travelling for life saving medical treatment, fly-in/fly-out miners and oil rig workers, newly-married honeymoon couples, someone who has saved every week for ten years for this holiday and can quote every word of the fine print in their well-thumbed holiday brochure.

And that catatonic lady over yonder. A first-time flier who is going to pick up the body of her dead son: killed on a motorcycle while on his gap-year holiday. There is one on just about every flight. Now you understand that tact and diplomacy of the cabin crew who, seeing "Bereaved Passenger" on the passenger manifest discretely move the middle aged lady into business class. Everyone's got a mother, and mothers aren't meant to outlive their kids.

It would be interesting to survey a plane load of people and discover their collective Holmes and Rahe Stress Scale ratings.

The *reason for the flight* is the main key to a good flight.

Maybe it would be better to use FedEx for the documents and spend money on video conferencing this trip, and save your flight for a relaxing holiday.

2. The Right Airline.

You can also sleep soundly by choosing the *right airline.*

Marketing departments would have you choose your airline by the color scheme, their advertising music, the catering and cabin crew experience. Seat pitch, the addition of business class bar or your own hotel suite in first or the quality of their movies. Not forgetting a restaurant style menu that was chosen by a television chef. What you *really* want to choose your airline by is its standard operating procedures, and the rigor to which those procedures are adhered.

You want spare parts that are purchased directly from the manufacturers, not from a "parts pooling" company where you are more likely to find counterfeit parts. With engineers who, in the middle of the night shift, are going to make the effort to get that tail-stand to double check that the top rudder bearings have been greased because they have pride in their work.

With pilots who are tested in the simulators at least twice a year.

Whose trained cabin crew have the latest communications with MedAire's Medlink[105] specialists in Arizona and all the required medical equipment, including a defibrillator, on board all of their flights. Remember, after a heart attack the chance of recovery without a defibrillator is about 2%. You need one to get you going again.

Whose every sector does *not* arrive at a hub in the middle of the Inter Tropical Convergence Zone, because you want to AVOID thunderstorms, not go where they breed.

These airlines cost money. But in reality the airfare is such a small component of your holiday; what do you care if the best airlines cost an extra $300 or $500? Pay the money, and get a cheaper hotel room. Why do you need such an expensive hotel anyway, you're only there to sleep?

The right airline has a good safety record.

If you are travelling for all the right reasons, and have discarded the concept of flying seven hours for less than the price of your taxi to the airport; now it's time to start planning by getting into the swing of things weeks ahead.

3. Passport

Ensure it is valid. Each country has rules before issuing visas. Most require that your passport is valid for six months from the date of entry.

4. Visas

Ensure there is enough room for the Visas in your passport. Countries with leaders who wear uniforms with tassels on their shoulders and a piece of rope tying their arm to their belt tend to demand a full page to apply their colorful visas. Lots of empty pages are needed for some holidays and some destinations require your passport a long time before the visa is approved.

A travel writer friend was not allowed onto an Air India flight at Shanghai that was transiting in Delhi because he did not have a visa for India. Even though he was doing nothing more than swapping onto a Sri Lankan Airlines flight in the terminal. No way in the world could he convince the Chinese check-in staff that he wouldn't swoon as soon as he saw Delhi from the air and decide to try to enter the country illegally.

(*'They've obviously never seen the pollution in Delhi,'* I told him. *'Everyone knows you can't see it until 200 feet before touchdown.'*)

His job? Travelling as a guest on Air India's new Boeing 787 to write a story about the new airplane. Have a guess how his review went since the plane took off without him? Never under estimate the number of people who arrive at a departure airport without the correct visas each day. Without them, we'd never get seats on staff travel. Triple check your visa.

5. Travel agent

For that reason alone, you cannot beat the worth of a good travel agent.

A large number of people have stuffed-up their own bookings on the internet. Twice now people have arrived at the airport of Sydney, Nova Scotia in Canada wondering if they can take a tour of the distinctive bridge and opera house. One guy interviewed on television said that he wondered when they got on a sixteen seater plane at Halifax; *'I thought Australia was more popular than this.'*

And thousands have realized, at the last second, TODAY is our return flight. *That bloody International Date Line gets you every time ...*

When you book with a travel agent, they cannot book you on flights which are inside the IATA transit connection limit. You and your baggage WILL connect. They arrange your itinerary, check your passport and arrange your visas. They have access to special discounts and hotel package deals AND cost you nothing. They get commission from the airlines.

But the best thing is that you can call them from check-in at an airport and ask them to arrange something. Within minutes you are relaxing in your seat and they are emailing confirmations, your credit card is on their record. On some carriers your updated e-tickets come straight to your phone in-flight. James Bond couldn't function without Miss Moneypenny. You can't function without a travel agent. Get a good one, and you'll keep them for life.

While you are planning your flights, think about airport transit hotels. Singapore has a great one, including a rooftop swimming pool. You can be in your room within ten minutes of exiting your plane, sleep restfully in the spartan but adequate room, then spend time up by the pool before your next flight. Capped-off by a foot massage, it can make breaking the trip worthwhile if, by using multiple carriers, you make substantial savings. Your travel agent can arrange the transit hotel bookings at the same time as you buy the tickets. Most big airports have them, but there are only a small number of rooms, so book early.

6. Earplugs and eye shades

Train yourself to use earplugs and eye shades. They don't call New York the city that never sleeps for nothing. At 3 a.m. on Sunday mornings, it's normal for taxi drivers to honk their horns at pedestrians crossing legally with total disregard for those trying to sleep above. And you have not lived until you have heard the never-ending thrum of Asian motorcycles outside your room. Whether you need them for your flights or your destination, it takes about two weeks to get used to sleeping with ear plugs and sleep masks. Start tonight.

7. Frequent flier

Go online and join the airline's frequent flier program NOW. Even if you make a temporary card made of paper, joining ensures that you start accruing points from the first sector. You may also be entitled to check-in privileges, airport lounges, and upgrades. All you need is a membership number for the computer.

Since the introduction of K-Class (computerized ticketing) in the 1990s, airlines consistently refine the sales offering to ensure that the planes are full. Starting two years out, when they open flights, passenger loadings are examined at various points on the time scale to see how they flight is filling. Fares are tweaked and promotions are added to attract the right numbers at the "gates" when the loads are examined (18 months out, 1 year, six months and so on).

Empty airline seats are worth nothing as soon as the door is closed, and the industry is distinctive in that, unless they bought tickets together, no passenger knows what the person sitting next to them has paid. Imagine opening a bakery on that premise? It's magic. It allows them to defeat the fickle nature of the general public who also cover themselves by double-booking on multiple flights, even other airlines, to make sure they can travel whenever it suits them. People travelling for business are happy to pay extra for fully flexible tickets, in case their meeting runs over or the client wants to go for a drink or dinner after then deal is done. Which means that the airline has no idea how many people are going to turn up on the day. Using historical data (this flight's loads will change based on day of the week if nothing else) they overbook Economy, on some flights up to 120%.

The passengers with money who the airline wishes to look after most of all are *not* always those traveling in First or Business whose tickets are paid by their company or the government. It's those small business people in the first few rows of Economy. Unlike the corporates who can get about 50% discount for bulk-buying, the small business person must have full flexibility, and is paying full retail.

Overbooking Economy allows the flight to go as full as possible. The airline knows that some people are going to miss their flight, others discover at check-in that they don't satisfy the ultimate destination's visa requirements, or that their passport is about to expire, or they have left it at home. Others arrived so early that the airline offered to put them on an earlier flight. The check-in process continues and people who matter to the airline's future, frequent fliers, are given upgrades into the next class of travel. By exposing them to the higher class it is hoped that, next time, they will buy the more expensive ticket. Business up into First, Economy into Business. Then, when the counters close only forty-five minutes to the flight, staff travel seats are used to fill up the plane if there is anything left. The golden days of staff travel are over.

That's why you join the Frequent Flier program. You're hoping that they have overbooked and you are there to help them out of a spot. But you have to look the part. If they have to upgrade someone and there are two options, the well-dressed person wins every time.

Which is why I have motto: *"There are only two places that miracles happen on a daily basis: Hospital Emergency Rooms and Airport Check-In Counters."* I am the only person who wears a smart suit every time I go on holiday, and I go out of my way to help the airline by being ready to assume a higher grade seat if they need.

8. Credit cards and airport lounge access

Read the fine print that comes with your credit card. In most cases, if you bought your air ticket with it you are entitled to free travel insurance. Their website will have the latest details.

Often credit cards entitle you to access airport lounges, say, five times a year. You can often put up with Economy on multiple sector trips, provided that you have access to the oasis that is an airport lounge during a stopover.

If you cannot get free lounge access with your ticket or credit card, check out the lounges at your planned airports by looking at each airport's website. You can also join lounge clubs and receive special treatment, (PriorityPass[106], Lounge Pass[107], and Lounge Club[108]). Large airports have lounge access where you pay on the day, but for some reason they try to keep it a secret on their websites. Get your eight-year-old niece to search your intended airports. She'll find it in seconds. Or look at *The Guide To Sleeping In Airports* website[109].

9. Travel insurance

If you don't think travel insurance can help you sleep adequately, try having a ski holiday in the U.S.A. without it. Medical bills can ruin your life, even if the injury is minor. You'd hate to remain behind in a third-world hospital after seeing your fellow survivor being airlifted out by medivac to Singapore for first-class treatment, because they had better insurance than you.

10. Meals, seats and online check-in.

Investigate the seating and meal options *no later* than a week before the flight. For some airlines the special meal cutoff may be two weeks out. SeatGuru.com[110] has configurations for all main airlines including reviews of the best and worst places to sit. Study your flight, know which type of aircraft you'll be catching and choose your seat. An aisle seat is preferable if you intend to roam the airplane. Excellent for a quick getaway, you can leave your finished meal tray in place and slide out.

Get friendly with your airline's frequent flier website. Fill in as much of your profile as you can. If your bladder can stand it, choose a window seat, midway from the noisy toilets and galley, as far away from the cabin bulkheads which will be the location of the on-board bassinets.

Since the special meals get served first, always book a special meal. The low fat or vegetarian options are acceptable. Your mission is to be served first, then use the bathroom first before retiring to watch a pre-sleep movie, before your fellow passengers. The state of the washrooms is going to deteriorate. (Unless you fly the airline with the showers in First Class. Their A380s have two diligent cabin service attendants who clean all the washrooms every half an hour.)

Two days before you fly set your alarms to make sure you are ready to click as soon as online check-in opens and grab your seat. Be aware that some flights actually commence in another city or country and your port is the stopover. If so, many seats will have gone already. Have a backup plan.

11. Audiobooks

Join Audible[111].com, buy twelve credits for whatever they charge, and choose about six books of varying tastes. You will be surprised how enjoyable waiting in lines, or in departure lounges, can become. Having already started a lengthy book before the flight will make it easier. Good luck with trying to remember all the names in the first hour of an Agatha Christie novel while negotiating an international airport.

12. Change the channel

Sleep better by not watching episodes of *Air Crash Investigation* in the lead-up to your flights. As they are repeated every few months you will be able to catch up when you get back home. Anyway, the reason for the crash on the episode you'll miss was fixed in 1983 and is unlikely to reoccur. *The reason for the crash in which you are going to die hasn't been discovered yet …*

13. Time travel

Start getting towards your new time zone. If your trip is going to involve a massive time zone shift, start moving your sleeping patterns towards your destination. About a week out, start being aware of its local time, set a clock in your house, maybe on the microwave. TuneIn Radio[112] allows you to begin listening to the local news and weather. PressReader.com[113] allows you to read their local newspapers.

14. Deal with the fear

Recognize (talking to non-Pilots here, I hope) if you have a slight fear of flying. This can affect your sleep patterns leading up to the flight, and throughout your entire career. In the weeks before you take off as a passenger you can work on these fears by getting educated about the *"Principles of Flight."* You will be in the minority of passengers on your flight who understands why you leave the earth.

Understanding that you are, more than likely, *a person who likes to be in control* (I didn't say control-freak) makes it easy to see why flying is an issue. It's this relinquishing of control to unseen people (and other cabin crew) that makes flying difficult. In the same way doctors make horrid patients, more than a few pilots are not very good passengers. Further research on the quality of training of the crews, and the highly supervised work of the engineers and air traffic controllers should also give you confidence.

Before 9/11 we used to have passengers sit in the jump seat to share the view of take-off and landing. The most fearful flyer was instantly cured as they felt part of the crew, with their headset on listening to ATC, and being able to see out the front. More than a few went on to become private pilots themselves.

Some airlines have magical in-flight video cameras, "pilot eye view" and even "tail cam" on the A380. Make sure you work out these controls as soon as you sit in your seat for the full wide-screen view (see if you can catch the tug driver sending SMS messages to his wife while waiting for the baggage loading to finish).

YouTube has some fantastic in-cockpit footage of take-off and landings. Search for *'FLYING TIARE - French Polynesia with a go pro - Air Tahiti Nui'*[114] celebrating the 15th birthday of the Air Tahiti's A340. It is captivating.

15. Socks

Buy some flight socks, the type that go at least to your knee and compress the lower leg and feet. They are designed to prevent Deep Vein Thrombosis. Having used them on long flights for a decade I can attest that you will arrive feeling "fresher." A pair of thick oversized hiking socks will also keep your feet warm while you sleep. If nothing else, the compression socks stop your feet swelling, making it easier to get your shoes back on as you reach the destination. Less-bendy people find slip-on shoes helpful for air travel.

16. Plan ahead

Much pre-flight sleep is lost by worrying about communication. Mobile phone coverage, roaming rates, internet access for email, and ensuring snail-mail is dealt with back home. Before you travel, join WhatsApp[115], the world's largest phone system. As long as you have Wi-Fi access, you can send and received texts for free. Not only texts but sound bites and pictures, even free calls in some countries. Check with your overseas friends to see if they also have WhatsApp. You may have to add a second version of their number, complete with country code, before the system finds them in your phone and loads them into the app.

Check with your phone provider. To save you incurring huge bills if your phone is stolen, some companies do not allow global roaming unless you advise them in writing beforehand. And without Wi-Fi at hand, you may need to make calls the minute you land.

Oh, and turn off data-roaming unless you are rich. Come to think of it, data-roaming can make rich people go broke. Leave it off. There's enough free Wi-Fi in the world for you. Or buy a local sim card for longer stays.

It's the same with credit cards. Start using your credit card in a foreign country, especially for small amounts (the way criminals check if the card works), and if you don't answer your bank's call to your home mobile within seconds you can be assured your card will be turned off. Some banks don't even ring. This is not the way to ensure relaxing sleep on the first night of your month-long vacation. As well as your phone company, contact your credit card help desk and advise them when and where you are travelling. It may be mandatory if you are expecting to use their travel insurance.

17. Doctor

It's hard to sleep in jail (so I am told); well, for the first few nights anyway. You could be headed for a long holiday in a small room if you take controlled drugs across a border. Quite a few countries have restrictions on medications that are widely available in other states. Codeine, cold tablets, anti-depressants and sleeping pills and others could land you in hot water. Get your doctor to write a letter detailing your prescriptions and medications, and you will sleep better. You may also need to update your vaccinations. Some countries need to see a vaccination booklet.

18. Nicotine

If you are a heavy smoker the alveoli in your lungs (the small sacs that transfer the oxygen into your blood) think you are already at about 8,000 feet above sea level. That's higher than where you'd be sleeping at nearly all ski resorts. By flying you add the cabin altitude and discover that your lungs are already above 15,000 feet, in the range for mild hypoxia. By law you need supplemental oxygen above 14,000 feet, but of course, you don't realize it.

Every person's reaction to hypoxia is different, and with you for life. Some people feel extremely happy, like they had three Mai-Tais on an empty stomach. Other people may become anxious or confused, short of breath, start coughing or wheezing, have a rapid heart rate, even a change in skin color. We've heard stories of people who have tried to open the aircraft doors at altitude, or demanded to see the captain. Some want to fight.

Pilots undertake "chamber runs" in aviation decompression chambers. They are instantly taken from sea level to 25,000 feet in a simulation of an explosive decompression to get hypoxia. There they are observed by a partner who is wearing an oxygen mask while they perform simple tasks: identifying cards, writing their name, doing simple math problems, drawing five-pointed stars and finishing by signing their name.

Within seconds their performance is amusing to their partner, after a minute to two they are told to put on their own oxygen mask. Most cannot. Their partner, sitting opposite, reaches over and affixes their mask and hits the 100% button. Immediately the victim's color returns and within seconds their faculties have resumed. Having discovered their own symptoms they know that if they ever feel that way again in an airplane, they have to dive for an oxygen mask to remain conscious.

Then the exercise is repeated for their partner and they assume the role of safety pilot. Mind-blowing, considering that minutes earlier they were effectively crippled. The recovery is total. Provided they get oxygen fast enough. YouTube has some impressive hypoxia demonstrations[116].

When a mild to heavy smoker is hypoxic, whose individual symptoms are "being belligerent," and hasn't had a cigarette for three hours, well let's just say, now you know why people smoke in aircraft toilets and pick fights with crew members. And when you hear that six other passengers piled on top of a passenger who tried to open a door in flight, you're getting the message.

Why don't airlines offer ALL passengers who are smokers free nicotine patches, or nicotine chewing gum, so they don't have to suffer withdrawals when we know that they are mildly hypoxic to start with? Wouldn't that be the ultimate in customer service? The answer is "because of the lawyers." Nicotine is a drug and airline staff cannot dish out drugs to passengers. Maybe one day Medlink doctors will, over the satellite phone, authorize crew to administer nicotine chewing gum, but it's doubtful.

If you are a smoker and plan a long flight, get a prescription from your doctor if needed, but don't get on that plane without nicotine patches or nicotine chewing gum to stop you climbing the walls. You'll sleep better. *And the crew won't have to restrain you.*

19. Pack cleverly

Even if you are going away for ten years, they **do** have shops overseas. Travel as light as you can. Choose outfits that can mix and match. Aim for lightweight clothes and put on a number of layers. Unless you are a full-fledged mountaineer, leave the backpack at home. Grab a daypack and then put it inside an expensive, lightweight, hard shell (bed bug resistant) suitcase that has good wheels and a name that starts with *Samson* and ends with *ite;* or, (according to my Editor) ends in *Tourister.*

Expect that your check-in luggage will go missing. Expect that your carry-on hand baggage will go missing.

In the old days it was wise to photocopy your passport, visas, credit cards, I.D. cards, (front and back) and hide them in the lining of your luggage and in your carry-on. Even a few Traveler's Checks *(remember them, Mr. Wong?)* You'd be grateful of them if you got mugged. I still hide a few hundred U.S. dollars emergency money, in case. If nothing else it makes a pleasant surprise five years later when you go away again. It can guarantee a Christmas card if you give your old suitcase to your niece.

These days though, an internet 'cloud' service like Evernote[117].com or DropBox[118].com is invaluable. Scans of every e-ticket, train, hotel and car rental booking, travel insurance details, doctor's letters, prescriptions, as well as all your cards and identity cards can leave your home computer, fly to the cloud, and simultaneously be available on your phone and iPad. Or from any computer in the world that you can use to log into their site. Make sure that, for your trip, your phone and iPad are security locked. And enable the "find my iPhone" option on all your devices.

Packing early and having all your documents secure can help you sleep well on the night before your trip. Few people get a good night's sleep before a flight, so are starting off at a disadvantage.

When you consider how many cranky, sleep-deprived people they have to deal with every day, it makes you respect the check-in staff; who are always grateful if you give them a packet of candies to share after the rush dies down.

20. Get there early

Say goodbye to your family and friends, defeat traffic and transportation snarls and head to the airport *very* early. This counts especially for Staff Travel. Get to the place where miracles happen early. Even if the seats aren't handed out until the last thirty minutes, the check-in staff will appreciate that you came out early to make their lives easier, will have had a chance to see that you are well-dressed, and may even make a mental note to bump you into a higher grade.

You will never get a seat on an overbooked airplane by sitting in a hotel room. Go to the airport, look fantastic, and be early. The sooner your bags are checked in and you are holding a boarding pass, the sooner you can relax.

21. Enjoy the airport

Since the 1990s lots of airports have been purchased by shopping center owners. No wonder considering that the top ten airports each see more than sixty million passengers a year, about 165,000 people each day. A captive market if ever there was one. With the added duty-free and fat holiday wallets, they have turned the concourses into shopper's delights using all the psychological tricks to attract buyers. Dubai Duty Free, servicing the seventy million passengers who pass through one of the world's largest international airports, turns over two billion dollars a year.

Treat yourself to the latest technology pocket-sized camera and a pair of in-ear earphones every time you go on holidays. Sunglasses, watches, and books seem to be mandatory purchases. (It's always confused me why they sell luggage *after* you have gone through security and customs. Does that guy ever make a sale?)

Expect that the air-conditioning in the airport will be a few degrees too hot. It is cheaper to keep it about 25 Celsius (77 Fahrenheit) instead of 18 Celsius (65 Fahrenheit), plus, you will be more stressed and hence, warmer than usual. This is why layers of loose-fitting clothing is required.

Depending on the ground air-conditioning, the aircraft may also be too warm until about ten minutes after departure when the aircraft air-conditioning has a chance to work effectively. Later during the flight, depending where you will be sitting, it could get cool. Wait until you have gone through security before buying a bottle of water or they will confiscate it from you. (Why? There are some explosives that can be made by mixing two clear liquids.) Once through security buy and keep drinking more water. Make sure you have a fresh bottle when you go onboard.

As well as shopping, your focus is walking, walking, and more walking. Same if you have a ninety-minute stopover. Walk, and keep walking until you are required for boarding. Buy some chocolates or barley sugar to "buy-off" your fellow passengers. You are never going to see them again, so while it's important to be polite, you have to manipulate them to allow you to sleep. Be first on, know where you are sitting, and grab your overhead space. Claim your seat and keep an eye on empty seats nearby. As fast as a striking snake you are going to steal another pillow as a lumbar support if possible. Try to do it so fast that no-one notices.

Keep standing and moving, then be pleasant to your arriving fellow travelers. As they settle, make small talk with them and the person beside you. Offer a chocolate or barley sugar. As soon as they have accepted, they are subconsciously thinking that you are a nice person and there is less chance that you are going to suffer armrest or seat-back warfare. The crew don't mind if you offer them a chocolate either. If you are on an aisle seat, explain before you sleep, (more chocolates), that we are all adults, and it's a matter of getting through this flight: *'If I am asleep and you need to get up and go for a walk, don't be precious, just clamber over me, OK?'* Chances are that they won't even wake you.

Buy a book but don't expect to read. Maybe it's mild hypoxia, but despite best intentions, most people struggle to read while airborne. Audiobooks are popular. If you fall asleep, you can wind them back, and the dulcet tones of the narrator can have a soothing effect.

Of course movies help pass the time, but the loud music and sound effects may tend to prevent sleep. If it is *Marley and Me* you can expect that a flight attendant will materialize to ask if you want anything as you are bursting into tears. Not giving away the ending here, but they stand behind you waiting for the moment. I am sure they do. Mild hypoxia makes grown men cry at the movies.

Time your arrival at the gate so that you don't need to sit with the masses. They will give a pre-boarding announcement for people with small kids. Ideally, you walk straight to the front of the line as others are hearing the boarding P.A. You don't want to breathe anyone's cold germs and airport boarding lounge air-conditioning is no-where near as effective as that on the aircraft.

22. On the aircraft

Inside the aircraft the air is admitted above your head and extracted at floor level (it is wise to position the gasper vent so as to provide a constant curtain of air). Theoretically you can't breathe air from anyone even one row in front or behind you. It passes through filters that are equivalent to (the manufacturer's say *better than*) the filters used in hospital operating theatres. A percentage flows into the cargo compartment and is exhausted overboard, and the rest is filtered again and mixed with fresh air from the front of the jet engines. The air in an A380 is changed every three minutes. The pilots can seal up cargo compartments and extract cabin air in case of smoke or fumes with the flick of a switch.

All the air in the toilets is, thankfully, extracted overboard.

The air, while being cleaned of 99% of the nasty germs, is low in humidity. It is around 12%, which is drier than normal. The only way to defeat the drying-out of your skin is to add moisturizer, and for your mucus to add water. Lots of ingested water. If you are feeling thirsty you are already dehydrated.

Contact germs, from touching surfaces and then your face and eyes, can be defeated by a hand sanitizer. Make sure that it is the 50ml bottle as 100 ml bottles may be confiscated by airport security. Wipes may be easier.

Move in your seat. Every twenty minutes or so move your feet, toes, and legs to get your blood flowing. Shrug your shoulders, twist and turn your neck. The adage of walking around the airplane is a nice concept, but impractical. Some people do it, and maybe it works for them. If the seatbelt sign is on and you are walking around, and the plane hits clear air turbulence, you can forget being compensated by the airline. If your flying body breaks a kid's neck, it could be the most expensive flight of your life.

The aisle-walkers would benefit more by staying in their seats, doing leg exercises, and learning to deep breathe. Hours breathing off the top of your lungs must add to the mild hypoxia. Whenever you think of it, try three huge deep breaths in a row, emptying your lungs, holding it, then filling your lungs to capacity, then a little more, and even more; hold it before repeating.

Sleeping on long flights can be assisted by knowing that your money and documents are secured in your cabin baggage in such a way that a quick thief opening the overhead bins would be foiled and move on to an easier mark. When you wake you should be able to reach out, without lifting your eye mask, grab your bottle, have a sip of water, then pop a barley sugar or chocolate in your mouth for a sugar hit, and drift back off to sleep.

23. The approach and landing

Arrange yourself so that your phone, wallet and passport are on your person before the approach and landing in case you have to do an emergency evacuation. Look at the emergency exits around you and make a note if you are going to go forward or back. The seats fold forward once their passengers have gone and jammed the aisle. Going forward beside the wall may be an option.

A documentary interviewed survivors from all sorts of disasters: tsunami, shipping disaster, air crash and building fire. Every victim had made a conscious decision that they were not going to die that day and reacted accordingly. When disaster strikes, it strikes hard, and you have to get tough or die. Have a plan.

Now we have covered the morbid side of landing; don't forget to watch the approach on TV if you can, especially from tail-cam if it is available. The pilot will be looking at the aiming point (the two big white boxes) in the middle of the touchdown zone. There are also some red and white lights next to it.

The touchdown zone is a box that extends to 900 meters (980 yards) down the runway. The large white boxes start 400 meters (440 yards) from the start of the runway. The manufacturer (and you) want the aircraft to be touching down inside the zone which, incidentally, is longer than the tallest man-made building is high. The runway is three or four kilometers (two to three miles) long, so you have heaps of margin.

As the pilot gets close to the touchdown zone, it is coming at them at 260 kph (160 mph). They switch their focal point to the end of the runway and start flaring the aircraft. You can see as the image tilts up. At the same time thrust is reduced. The wings squash the air trapped between them and the runway, like balloons, and the plane settles onto the ground.

If the wind is coming from the side they will crab along the center line then, in the flare, squeeze the rudder (with foot pedals) to point the nose down the runway. With a tiny flick of the wrist they will put the main wheel on the windward side onto the ground first, then the other side, and then the nose.

If the runway is contaminated they'll go for a "positive touchdown" to ensure the rubber of the wheels gets through the slush onto the runway.

As soon as the mains go on, the top of the wings open up. This dumps all the lift and puts the weight onto the wheels which allows the brakes to work efficiently. They may also select reverse thrust, although it is not needed unless the runways are contaminated. If you can see the engines you will see the sides open up. The exhaust which had been going out the back will now be directed forward. It's effective at high speed, and these will be stowed by 140 kph (85 mph) so they don't kick up debris which could then get sucked into the front of the engines.

Relax and go with it.

If your great-grandfather could see you now, he'd be jealous. Mankind has waited centuries to do what you are doing.

And you're doing it without even messing up your hair.

RECAPPING:

- Make sure you're flying for the right reasons, if you can.
- Choose a safe airline.
- Make sure passports and visas are correct.
- Use a travel agent.
- Start using earplugs and eye shades.
- Join the frequent flier programs of your intended flights.
- Credit cards.
- Travel insurance.
- Meals and Seats.
- Buy Audiobooks.
- Turn off air crash channels.
- Time travel.
- Deal with the fear.
- Plan ahead.
- Get compression socks.
- See your doctor about your drugs.
- If you smoke, get nicotine gum or patches.
- Pack cleverly.
- Get there early, go through security.
- After security, buy hand sanitizer, water, and chocolates.
- Walk, Walk, Walk.
- On board, greet your fellow passengers.
- Make sure they can't steal your goodies.
- Keep valuables close during takeoff and landing.
- Enjoy the experience.

From the Logbook

Why I love Travel Agents #1:

My Bristol travel agent booked me on the Eurostar from London to Paris. A special deal gave me a hotel room for 95 euros a night. Deciding to stay an extra night I went downstairs and tried to extend.

'Mon plaisir!' the happy receptionist beamed, *'... for an extra 390 Euros.'*

The 95 euro deal was most certainly only for travel agents.

I emailed my travel agent and within five minutes he faxed the hotel. The receptionist then extended me for 95 euros.

Why I love Travel Agents #2:

At check-in after a twelve hour transit at Hong Kong, a Cathay check-in lady demanded to charge excess baggage. I called my Bahraini travel agent and asked him to clarify my ticket conditions to the Cathay lady, who was trying to raise money to buy a new aircraft, then handed her the phone. I have no idea what he said but she smiled, apologized and processed my ticket, no extra charge.

And Finally ...

There you have it. Congratulations for having arrived here, at the end, of "Sleeping for Pilots & Cabin Crew, (And Other Insomniacs)."

Most people don't realize how hard it is for flight crew to sit and read a book that isn't a work manual, official company notice or change to procedures. Really. *Why should I waste time on my day off to read about a new type of passenger personal medical oxygen generator?* Instead we tend to survive on magazines, surfing the web and audiobooks for pleasure, and only pull out the written word when preparing for simulators and emergency revalidation.

Except in this case. So I thank you.

We have seen that there are things that can affect the amount and quality of sleep we get; most sleep-aids are a waste of money, and we have discovered that short-term fixes aren't going to help us in our long career. Our sleep is different to other workers. Everyone else gets a roster with a similar sign-on time for five days in a row. They mightn't like the sign-on time, but it allows adjustment. Our *"early start one day, late finish the next"* is unique to the flight crews of airliners. And you have a right to bitch and moan about your sleep, or the lack of it.

Good luck staying in a relationship with someone like my mate, Karim, at the pool. If they don't understand your work and sleep cycles then you have no chance. When you find someone who does, marry them. *Then make them tiptoe around the house with the TV and phone turned down.*

What we have learned from this book is you have to put your sleep above all else and plan your rest in advance. Get control of your life so that you can trick your brain, when needed, and take advantage of your ninety minute sleep cycle in order to get into that deep, restorative, rapid eye movement sleep. And wake up naturally, before the noisy alarms go off.

We now understand that 90% of getting a good sleep in a hotel room, or any room, is feeling safe and comfortable. Once your subconscious is satisfied, and your brain emptied, only then will it let you sleep. Get with the program, satisfy it, and stop faffing-around. We have seen how having a positive attitude at work can help make those long night flights whizz by, and make you feel good about yourself. Which leads to getting to sleep easier.

Because that's what it's all about, isn't it?

Those ten minutes after the light goes out.

'The only thing you ever do, where you have to
  ***pretend you're doing it** ... in order to do it.'*

You have become someone who works on airplanes, AND can sleep at will. You are one in a million.

Good night.

What's Next?

If you have enjoyed this book I would be grateful if you would go to this book's Amazon's page and give me an honest review.

[Amazon.com and search Sleeping Pilots … it always finds me]

An author's life is a solitary one, tapping keys in the silence, and reviews on the Amazon site are the reward for all the work. The more reviews from locations all around the world, the more people will buy the book. It's that simple. It's the new word-of-mouth. It's what authors live for.

My dream is to get onto the best-seller lists which can help a book to "breakout" from the masses and gain real attention. Your book review will *really* help me.

If you would like to recommend it on your social media, that'd be great too, and get your friends to click to the website and sign-up for the free Bonus Chapter, which will help them suffer those long haul flights as a passenger.

Hopefully, the more we can spread the word the more people will get a handle on how to sleep effectively, and will start to enjoy their airline life, instead of being worn-out by it.

With a bit of work and planning you can build a great career in this vibrant, young industry. Unlike many traditional businesses, women have the same chances as men, and are paid the same. Peoples' sexuality is not an issue and you're given a job based on what you can do for the company in the future, not for what you've done in the past.

In that respect alone, our industry is light years ahead of everyone else.

I really value your feedback, to hear how the tips have worked for you and to hear if you have any other sure-fire winners for further editions.

Have a look at our website:
www.ProfessionalSleeping.com
We made it just for you.

Feel free to email me at:
contact@professionalsleeping.com
depending on my roster (and sleep cycles),
I will get back to you as fast as I can.

Acknowledgements

I was about to get carried away and mention all the people who have helped get this book into your hands, then I realized that I am *Anonymous* and not allowed to mention who I am, or who I work for.

That's something about this business that I can understand, but don't like. Signing an employment contract which is also a confidentiality agreement makes sense ... especially after an inevitable crash. They can't have the families of the passengers bombarded by hundreds of opinions in the media. So the lawyers and accountants micro-manage the business and it all seems a little sterile.

Meanwhile we, who have the knowledge, experience and considered opinions, have to sit and watch rent-a-mouth private pilots on the television talking about our business as if they have a clue.

That sound you can hear on the wind? That's us yelling at the idiot *"Retired Air Force Colonel"* on Fuxed News telling the audience that Malaysian's 777 was *'stolen by the Pakistanis'*.

Anyone with any aviation experience knows that the border between India and Pakistan is the second-most sensitive border in the world. There ain't no way that 777 went that-a-way without being challenged.

Here I acknowledge my employer who approved my writing a previous book under my own name and who, despite requesting anonymity, wished me luck with this one.

And to all my family and friends who have put up with my pontificating on this, and many other subjects for many years.

To my work colleagues, whose inability to stay awake on the shortest of flights inspired me to commit my learned tips and tricks to paper.

To **Mark Baker**, and all the Flight Engineers I have ever flown-with, who gave me the tips to start with.

To those who inspired me to fly and to every one who I have flown with, pilots and cabin crew. I have learnt something new every day, and had a ball doing it.

To **Dr. Joe Loftus**, whose simple trick to knock-off bed bugs (and other crawlies) will help us all.

To **Lorelou Desjardins**, (the Frog in the Fjord), **Navjot Singh, Michael Blamey, Dani Moger** and anyone else who answered my questions and steered me right … (or wrong) even **Karim** by the pool.

To my production team who works when I sleep:

Anthony Shawon - elite PhotoShop guru in Bangladesh who took my images of my watch and digital clock numbers and made etching magic for my front cover.

Nichole Moser - Editor extraordinaire in Canada who was very tough. Besides being powered-by-coffee, is the only person I know who, (she says), can sleep with a pillow between her knees. She started with draft #4. This is #22. We have 19 more books to do.

Luis Tellez - 3D image bender in Mexico who took my book cover and put it in the hands of the blonde girl for the website pics.

Bookclaw.com - the book design team in Croatia who turned text into a book and inspired me to learn how to do it myself so I could do the final tweak.

No book would be complete without an army of proof readers, in this case the twentieth draft was fixed by **Navjot Singh**, freelancing in London, **Ian Hunt** on his yacht in Canada, **Jenny Cole** in her rally car in Australia, **Doreen Newman** in her little plane in Moorabbin and **Cheryl Mayhew** high over the Indian Ocean.

Olwyn Jones, you are right … the U.S. English (chosen purely to satisfy the largest market) jars the flow for those of us from U.K, Australia and New Zealand. If the book breaks out, you'll get your own edition, promise.

To **female pilots**, I have used the male term 'he' when referring to pilots in this book. In all cases it is describing a pilot who is deficient in some form, so I thought I'd leave it at that. I apologize if you are offended and seek your forgiveness. I can make you deficient in a future edition if you wish. Having flown with female pilots for twenty four years now I figure it's a non-issue. You have just as much right to my seat as anyone else.

And, finally, **to all my passengers** who have paid real money so I can roll out onto the stage that is runway 27 right at Heathrow.

From controllers, ground staff, other pilots, fire-ies, to anoraks (plane spotters); the entire airport pauses, then stares enthralled as I charge down that strip of bitumen like Jeremy Clarkson on crack cocaine[##].

To rotate an A380 on takeoff and blast over London, when he'd be applying the brakes, is to have the time of your life![*]

Thank you all,

j.c.n.

[*]**Clive James** said of the Boeing 747:

"Unless you had been told, you would never think of it as having 400 people on board. It looks as if there is only one man in there, having the time of his life."

[##] In no way am I implying that Mr.Clarkson has ever used, or would ever use, crack cocaine. That we all can imagine how fast he'd drive in such a state, and how much fun it would be to watch, is a testament to his abilities and showmanship.

Endnotes

[1] Mayo Clinic
http://www.mayoclinic.org/

[2] Harvard Health
http://www.health.harvard.edu/

[3] Unicef http://www.unicef.org/

[4] World Health Organization
http://www.who.int/en/

[5] WebMD
http://www.webmd.com/

[6] Drugs.com
http://www.drugs.com/

[7] Wikipedia
https://en.wikipedia.org/wiki/Main_Page

[8] Google Scholar
https://scholar.google.com/

[9] New York City's Bed bug Webpage
http://www.nyc.gov/html/doh/bedbugs/html/home/home.shtml

[10] New York City's Bed bug Webpage
http://www.nyc.gov/html/doh/bedbugs/html/home/home.shtml

[11] Tips for Pooping Better
http://www.paulcheksblog.com/tips-for-pooping-better/

[12] Docs Say Stop Taking Multivitamins
http://healthland.time.com/2013/12/17/docs-say-stop-taking-multivitamins/

[13] Annals of Internal Medicine study of supplemental vitamins
http://annals.org/article.aspx?articleid=1789253

[14] Navjot Singh's website
http://www.navjot-singh.com/

[15] Mayo Clinic
http://www.mayoclinic.org/healthy-lifestyle/nutrition-and-healthy-eating/in-depth/caffeine/art-20045678

[16] WebMD
http://www.webmd.com/food-recipes/20150311/coffee-health-faq

[17] Ice Addict Rehabilitation
http://www.queendom.com/advices/advice.htm?advice=291

[18] Stilnox (Zolpidem)
https://en.wikipedia.org/wiki/Zolpidem

[19] iPetitions.com - Ban Stilnox, Imovane and related sleep medications

http://www.ipetitions.com/petition/stilnox/

[20] Mamamia Website: 'Stilnox Killed My Sister'
http://www.mamamia.com.au/news/stilnox-killed-my-sister

[21] The Royal Canadian Air Force 5BX exercise system for men.
http://csclub.uwaterloo.ca/~rfburger/5bx-plan.pdf

The Royal Canadian Air Force 10BX exercise system for women.
https://en.wikipedia.org/wiki/XBX Find the XBX Plan then download the
zipped file, unzip it and print.

[22] Audible.com
http://www.audible.com/

[23] Absolute Sleep Music
Good sleep music including my favorite, "Rain Sounds for Sleep and
Relaxation"
http://www.rhapsody.com/artist/absolute-sleep-music

[24] Sleep Phones, headphones in a headband.
http://www.sleepphones.com/

[25] Malaria Vaccine Org - "In the last hundred years more American
soldiers have become casualties of **mosquitoes** than **bullets**"
http://www.malariavaccine.org/files/FS_Malaria-Military_9-15-04.pdf

[26] Mosquito Facts
http://www.control-mosquitoes.com/

[27] The deadliest animal in the world by far
http://www.smithsonianmag.com/smart-news/mosquitoes-kill-more-
humans-human-murderers-do-180951272/

[28] Malaria
http://www.who.int/mediacentre/factsheets/fs094/en/

[29] Article written by Steven J. Lloyd and originally published in the June 2002 issue of *Vietnam* Magazine
http://www.historynet.com/us-vietnam-war-soldiers-and-malaria.htm

[30] The BBQ Stopper

http://www.abc.net.au/radionational/programs/backgroundbriefing/2014-01-28/5217856

[31] Chickungunya
http://www.who.int/mediacentre/factsheets/fs327/en/

[32] Woman Loses Vision after Mosquito Bites
http://www.livescience.com/51790-chikungunya-eye-problems.html

[33] Dengue Fever
http://www.betterhealth.vic.gov.au/bhcv2/bhcarticles.nsf/pages/Dengue_fever?open

[34] Ross River Virus
http://www.betterhealth.vic.gov.au/bhcv2/bhcarticles.nsf/pages/Ross_River_disease

[35] Murray Valley Encephalitis
http://www.betterhealth.vic.gov.au/bhcv2/bhcarticles.nsf/pages/Murray_Valley_encephalitis?open

[36] Yellow Fever
http://www.who.int/mediacentre/factsheets/fs100/en/

[37] West Nile Virus
http://www.betterhealth.vic.gov.au/bhcv2/bhcarticles.nsf/pages/West_Nile_virus?open

[38] U.S Soldiers and Malaria
http://www.historynet.com/us-vietnam-war-soldiers-and-malaria.htm

[39] What it feels like to have Malaria
http://www.nothingbutnets.net/blogs/what-it-feels-like-to-have-malaria.html?referrer=https://www.google.ae/

[40] 10 Ways to Guarantee You'll Get Mosquito Bites
http://insects.about.com/od/flies/a/how-to-get-mosquito-bites.htm

[41] Mosquito Nets
http://www.mosquitonets.com/

[42] Michael Blamey
http://www.michaelblamey.com/

43 Melatonin.
Brent A. Bauer, M.D
http://www.mayoclinic.org/melatonin-side-effects/expert-answers/
faq-20057874

44 Valerian.
http://www.drugs.com/mtm/valerian.html

45 Valerian.
http://www.mayoclinic.org/diseases-conditions/insomnia/expert-
answers/valerian/faq-20057875

46 Tony H. giving a talk.
Alcoholics Anonymous speech by Tony H.
https://www.youtube.com/watch?v=7sg1L2ysRqc

47 USA - Guide To Quitting Smoking
*http://www.cancer.org/%20healthy/stayawayfromtobacco/
guidetoquittingsmoking/index*

48 USA - How To Quit Smoking
http://www.helpguide.org/articles/addiction/how-to-quit-smoking.htm

49 UK - NHS Smoke Free
http://www.nhs.uk/smokefree

50 Australia - The Quit Organization
http://www.quit.org.au/

51 Tony H. giving a talk.
Alcoholics Anonymous speech by Tony H.
https://www.youtube.com/watch?v=7sg1L2ysRqc

52 Alcoholics Anonymous speech by Buzz A.
https://www.youtube.com/watch?v=R_nZBUUiltI

53 Passion Planner
www.passionplanner.com

54 WebMD
http://www.webmd.com/sleep-disorders/tc/snoring-cause

55 Snoring Partners - The Daily Mail
http://www.dailymail.co.uk/femail/article-2600997/Chin-straps-mouth-
shut-A-wristband-gives-electric-shocks-They-BOTH-snore-sleep-
starved-couple-cure.html

56 Mayo Clinic
http://www.mayoclinic.org/diseases-conditions/snoring/basics/definition/con-20031874

57 Body Mass Index Calculator
http://www.nhlbi.nih.gov/health/educational/lose_wt/BMI/bmi-m.htm

58 Koala's mating call
https://www.youtube.com/watch?v=BMXBV9oLbVk

59 Men's Health Tips
http://www.mens-health-tips.com/tips-to-stop-snoring.html

60 Mayo Clinic
http://www.mayoclinic.org/diseases-conditions/sleep-apnea/basics/definition/con-20020286

61 WebMd
http://www.webmd.com/sleep-disorders/sleep-apnea/

62 Men's Health Tips
http://www.mens-health-tips.com/tips-to-stop-snoring.html

63 Nytol Spray
http://nytol.co.uk/stop-snoring/

64 See what a CPAP machine looks like
http://www.resmed.com/ap/en/index.html

65 The Provent nostril plugs
http://www.proventtherapy.com

66 MindTools website:
http://www.mindtools.com/pages/article/newTCS_82.htm

67 Ozone Hole Repair
http://www.dailymail.co.uk/sciencetech/article-2753148/Ozone-layer-track-repair-says-scientists-Shield-protects-Earth-Sun-shows-early-signs-recovery.html

68 *Be Sun Smart*
http://www.sunsmart.com.au/

69 Skin Cancer & Sunlight
http://www.ccohs.ca/oshanswers/diseases/skin_cancer.html

[70] *A Frog in the Fjord* - Lorelou Desjardins' hilarious website, in particular: "How to survive your winter depression"
http://afroginthefjord.com/2013/12/08/how-to-survive-your-winter-depression/

[71] Dr. Erin S. LeBlanc's Vitamin D Study from the Center for Health Research, Kaiser Permanente Northwest, Pacific Northwest Evidence-based Practice Center, Oregon Health & Science University, Portland, Oregon, U.S.A.
http://annals.org/article.aspx?articleid=1938934

[72] Mind Body Green's "10 Reasons Why You Should Drink More Water"
http://www.mindbodygreen.com/0-4287/10-Reasons-Why-You-Should-Drink-More-Water.html

[73] NPR's expose: "How Much Water Actually Goes Into Making A Bottle Of Water?"
http://www.npr.org/sections/thesalt/2013/10/28/241419373/how-much-water-actually-goes-into-making-a-bottle-of-water

[74] UNICEF's "Water, Sanitation and Hygiene (WASH)" initiative
http://www.unicef.org/media/media_45481.html

[75] Water Initiative
http://www.thewaterinitiative.com

[76] "Abundance: The Future Is Better than You Think" (Audiobook)
http://www.audible.com/pd/Science-Technology/Abundance-Audiobook/B007OQ0MY2/ref=a_search_c4_1_2_srTtl?qid=1446467160&sr=1-2

[77] "Abundance: The Future Is Better than You Think" (Amazon Printed Book)
http://www.amazon.com/Abundance-Future-Better-Than-Think/dp/145161683X/ref=sr_1_1?ie=UTF8&qid=1446467067&sr=8-1&keywords=abundance+book

[78] BBC report on University Of Bristol's "Obesity linked to lack of sleep"
http://news.bbc.co.uk/2/hi/health/4073897.stm

[79] USA Today reported on a Columbia University study
http://usatoday30.usatoday.com/news/health/2004-12-06-sleep-weight-gain_x.htm

[80] WebMD Sleep More to Fight Obesity
http://www.webmd.com/diet/20041116/sleep-more-to-fight-obesity

[81] Kaiser Permanente Study "Sleep More to Fight Obesity"
http://www.kpchr.org/research/public/News.aspx?NewsID=62

82 Air India Grounds Crew
http://www.telegraph.co.uk/travel/travelnews/11863390/Air-Indias-flight-attendants-too-fat-to-fly.html

83 PreventDisease.com "16 Reasons To Have Daily Sex"
http://preventdisease.com/news/12/123012_16-Reasons-To-Have-Daily-Sex.shtml

84 Mr.Goh Choon Phong, CEO Singapore Airlines, Cover story interview
Airline Business Magazine - Jul-Aug 2015 Issue
http://www.flightglobal.com/interviews/year/15/goh-choon-phong/singapore-girl/

85 Weather Underground
http://www.wunderground.com/

86 Google
http://www.google.com

87 Low Blue Lights
https://www.lowbluelights.com/index.asp?

88 Hibermate Sleep Masks
http://www.hibermate.com/

89 Mayo Clinic's Slide Show to prevent back pain
http://www.mayoclinic.org/healthy-lifestyle/adult-health/multimedia/back-pain/sls-20076265

90 Napoleon Hill's   *"Think and Grow Rich"*

Amazon
http://www.amazon.com/Think-Grow-Rich-Original-Unedited/dp/193764135X/ref=sr_1_1?
ie=UTF8&qid=1438281717&sr=8-1&keywords=Napoleon+Hill%E2%80%99s+++%09+++++%E2%80%9CThink+And+Grow+Rich%E2%80%9D

Audible
http://www.audible.com/pd/Self-Development/Think-and-Grow-Rich-1937-Edition-Audiobook/B00OTZ6056/
ref=a_search_c4_1_8_srTtl?qid=1438282123&sr=1-8

91 Napoleon Hill's Rise & Fall
http://www.success.com/article/rich-man-poor-man

[92] Dale Carnegie's *"How to Win Friends and Influence People"*

Amazon
http://www.amazon.com/How-Win-Friends-Influence-People/dp/
B008GAT3BI/ref=sr_1_1?
ie=UTF8&qid=1438282617&sr=8-1&keywords=How+to+Win+Friends+
%26+Influence+People

Audible
http://www.audible.com/pd/Business/How-to-Win-Friends-Influence-
People-Audiobook/B002V5BV96/ref=a_search_c4_1_1_srTtl?
qid=1438282379&sr=1-1

[93] *Maxwell Maltz's "The New Psycho-Cybernetics"*

Amazon
http://www.amazon.com/Psycho-Cybernetics-New-More-Living-Life/dp/
0671700758/ref=sr_1_1?
ie=UTF8&qid=1438282787&sr=8-1&keywords=Psycho-Cybernetics
(A revamped edition is due out in November 2015)

Audible
http://www.audible.com/pd/Business/The-New-Psycho-Cybernetics-
Audiobook/B002UZMTN4/ref=a_search_c4_1_1_srTtl?
qid=1438283103&sr=1-1

[94] Zig Ziglar's *"See You at the Top"*
Amazon
http://www.amazon.com/See-You-Top-Anniversary-Hardcover/dp/
B00ZLWSTPK/ref=sr_1_2?
ie=UTF8&qid=1438283331&sr=8-2&keywords=See+You+at+the+Top
%3A+25th+Anniversary+Edition

Audiobook (lecture)
http://www.audible.com/pd/Business/See-You-at-the-Top-Audiobook/
B00AFH71VO/ref=a_search_c4_1_1_srTtl?qid=1438283175&sr=1-1

[95] Time Article on the NASA Nap and ATCs
http://swampland.time.com/2011/04/26/memo-to-the-boss-naps-
increase-performance/

[96] Improving alertness and performance in emergency department
physicians and nurses: the use of planned naps.
http://www.ncbi.nlm.nih.gov/pubmed/17052562

97 Cambridge University: Daytime Nappers Die Younger
http://www.medicaldaily.com/daytime-napping-may-lead-early-death-its-most-likely-sign-something-more-serious-276372

98 The new Napwell Mask
http://napwell.com/

99 Sebastian Reyes survives a 17 story fall
http://www.telegraph.co.uk/news/worldnews/southamerica/chile/11773154/Man-survives-fall-from-17th-floor-balcony-in-Chile-CCTV.html

100 Witopia Virtual Private Network
https://www.witopia.com/

101 TuneIn Radio
App for Apple and Android

102 PressDisplay and PressReader
http://www.pressdisplay.com
http://www.pressreader.com/

103 WhatsApp
http://www.whatsapp.com/

104 The New York Times reported that the American National Institute of Mental Health had put the number of Americans who suffered 'aviophobia' at 6.5%
http://www.nytimes.com/2007/07/24/health/psychology/24fear.html?_r=0

105 MedAire's Medlink In-Flight Medical Assistance
http://www.medaire.com/solutions/airlines/resource-center/in-flight-medical-events

106 PriorityPass Airport Lounges
http://www.prioritypass.com/

107 Lounge Pass Airport Lounges
https://www.loungepass.com/index.cfm?fuseaction=home.home

108 Lounge Club Airport Lounges
https://www.loungeclub.com

109 The Guide to Sleeping in Airports
http://www.sleepinginairports.net/airport-lounges/

110 Seat Guru
http://www.seatguru.com/

[111] Audible.com
http://www.audible.com/

[112] TuneIn Radio
App for Apple and Android

[113] PressDisplay and PressReader
http://www.pressdisplay.com
http://www.pressreader.com/

[114] Flying Tiare's stunning inflight footage
https://www.youtube.com/watch?v=P7EP9Ko6IsY

[115] Whatsapp
http://www.whatsapp.com/

[116] Hypoxia Chamber Run
https://www.youtube.com/watch?v=UN3W4d-5RPo

[117] Evernote.com
https://evernote.com/

[118] Dropbox.com
https://www.dropbox.com/